*Intermittent Fasting For Women: The 30 Day Whole Foods Adventure Lose Up to 30 Pounds Within A Month!*

*The Ultimate 30 Day Diet to Burn Body Fat. Your Weight Loss Surgery Alternative!*

responsible for any losses, direct or indirect, which are incurred as a result of the use of information contained within this document, including, but not limited to, —errors, omissions, or inaccuracies.

*Introduction....5*

*Chapter 1: What is Intermittent Fasting?....14*

*Chapter 2: Chronic Degenerative Diseases & Unhealthy Living.......79*

*Chapter 3: Why Wholefoods Are Beneficial?.....96*

*Chapter 4: Identify Your Body Type.... 113*

*Chapter 5: 30 Whole Foods & Recipes....123*

*Chapter 6: Conclusion....165*

## *Introduction*

This book is going to change your life! I know you just started reading, but I'm serious! My book is designed to impact your life in the most positive way possible from a holistic standpoint.

You probably decided to buy this book because you want to become a better version of yourself! You made the best investment to invest in your health and wellness. I got good news for you, and that is your life will be transformed once you start taking action and implementing these strategies I discuss within this book.

Are you tired of being bombarded by countless infomercials that endorse new diet fads? I'm pretty sure you've heard it all from, ketogenic diet, paleo diet, vegan diet and even the raw food diet. Now I'm not criticizing  or taking jabs at any of these mentioned diets, and I do truly believe in most cases these diets do work effectively to a certain degree.

But you see there lies an inherent problem with all these so called "diets". People tend to go on them and start seeing some results, but before you know it they start gaining back those unwanted pounds simply because they couldn't uphold their regiment. To add insult to injury a lot of these diets tend to be more costly and run a expensive bill that cannot be sustained on the average working person's budget.

Well, I'm here to tell you that intermittent fasting won't cost you anymore than you are already spending. This diet in particular is designed to help you burn unwanted body fat fast and sculpt your way to your ideal physique in conjunction to exercise.

But, before we start discussing the basics we need to get your mindset right! Something not discussed a lot within the health and fitness industry and that is having a good sense of self-awareness before you start any diet. You see the inherent problem I previously mentioned with all these diets is that people cannot uphold or continue on with certain diet regiments.

Why? Because people treat diets like prescription drugs! Once results are derived and an outcome is finalized people tend to go back to their old ways of living and relegate their newfound diet fad to the back burner.

You see there is an inherent problem when you interface with a diet and consider it a short term fix. True transformation takes place from the inside out and when you become aware changing the way you eat is not a matter of going on a short term diet, but a total lifestyle change!

That's right you need to transform your lifestyle or modify it in order to achieve long term sustainable results! You need to incorporate intermittent fasting as apart of your daily living, and in order to do this you need to shift your short term thinking to long term.- This is not a prescription drug.

### Obesity Epidemic – In Industrialized Societies

Studies have revealed that people found in the industrialized world (first world countries), in particular here in North America have extremely high obesity rates. *The Journal of the American Medical Association (JAMA)* estimates that nearly **35.5%** of women living in America are obese.

This rate has grown considerably over the past few years especially ever since the advent of instant foods, fast foods, refined carbohydrates and of course sugary drinks, pastries and other snacks.

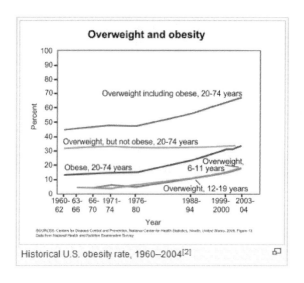

*Figure 1*

*Figure 1* displays historical data in the US showing constant increase and linear progression of the obesity epidemic that has plagued America. As you can see not even children are immune to obesity, but have easily become susceptible to excess fat because of poor lifestyle choices, despite having faster metabolisms.

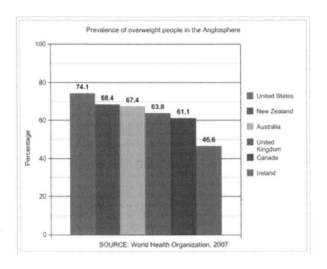

*Figure 2*

*Figure 2* shows obesity rates among English speaking nations and interestingly enough America ranks highest followed by New Zealand. Notice all the countries listed are industrialized and practice advanced agriculture including the manipulation of refined carbohydrates which is when foods are stripped of there fiber content, minerals, essential fats and vitamins in order to sustain a longer shelf-life.

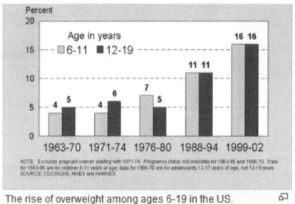

Percent

Age in years
□ 6-11  ■ 12-19

The rise of overweight among ages 6-19 in the US.

## *Figure 3*

*Figure 3* displays the prevalence of obesity among children ages 6-19. As you can see not even children can escape the consequences of poor lifestyle choices. You can see an increase of obesity rates from 1960s – below 5% of the population was obese, and from 1999 to the early 2000s over 15% of the population struggled with obesity. Now these are some disturbing statistics, it was bad enough that adults struggled with being overweight, but now even our children face the same problems. Not only that but children are now being diagnosed with "adult onset diseases" which have a strong correlation with obesity.

Now, I talked a lot about obesity rates among children and adults in most industrialized English speaking countries tend to be abnormally high, and you know the reasons behind obesity stem from poor lifestyle choices including lack of exercise and "Frankenstein foods".

But now let's do some compare and contrast, do you know which **industrialized** country has the lowest obesity rate and why? The answer is *Japan*! – That's right a country that boasts as one of the world's leading technological powerhouses with advanced technology, relatively low crime rates, fast transportation and let's not *forget quality food*!

So why do the Japanese have a much lower obesity rate in comparison to any other country of the industrialized parts of the world? The answer is simple, and that is their source of food! Japanese traditionally consume a lot of whole foods, while their counter parts the Americans eat foods that are heavily processed. It must be noted that American influence on Japanese cuisine is starting to infect Japanese people, but as a whole and generally speaking the Japanese eat much cleaner.

Have you ever stopped to consider one of their most iconic foods, sushi? You can easily break down what traditional sushi is made up of; rice, raw fish or cooked fish, and seaweed. You can easily identify the components part by part and this is what constitutes wholefoods!

Traditional sushi is made up of whole food ingredients, unlike our standard American "Frankenstein foods" that contain fillers, additives, preservatives and artificial sweeteners. This simple, but profound truth infers quite a lot. The fact is we need to start looking at our diets more closely and identify fake foods from authentic wholefoods.

The correlation between their low obesity rate and consumption of whole foods is indisputable. Not only are whole foods packed with dense calories, but contain the essential vitamins, minerals, fibers, and other nutritional benefits that all human beings need to survive.

Whole foods are plant based foods that have little to minimal processing and have not undergone any acritical alterations.

Obesity is a serious thing. Obesity can be considered a jumping off point to various chronic degenerative diseases. Hence, why its important to lose those unwanted pounds as quickly as possible. When you become overweight you're at risk to a plethora of chronic disease states, such as cancer, diabetes, high blood pressure, stroke, gout, and even arthritis.

The dangers of obesity and being overweight cannot be understated and I hope I was able to give you a quick summary in this introduction to why you need to lose those unwanted pounds as being overweight posses certain health risks and complications that not only effect your self-esteem and body image, but the outcome of your overall health too!

## Chapter 1:What is Intermittent Fasting?

Is intermittent fasting some new health fad that is taking the fitness industry by storm or is there more to it than meets the eye? What if I told you intermittent fasting isn't really something new!? – But people have been practicing it since ancient times! That's right our ancestors didn't have supermarkets, fast food restaurant chains, or any other sources of quickly accessible food, and thus as a result were forced to interface with intermittent fasting on a daily basis.

Food was scantly available and people didn't have the luxury of eating out on a whim or eating at their leisure. For a matter of fact a point I wanted to highlight is people didn't eat out of boredom like we do today! – Human beings are the only creatures on planet earth who eat out of boredom! Animals don't even do it!

Have you ever seen on wildlife documentaries prey such as buffalo or deer walking past content lions? Why don't the lions attack when they are content and their bellies are filled? This is not a strange phenomena, but a simple fact of life and that is animals only eat when they're hungry!- Not out of boredom.

Human beings have acquired the habit of eating for either out of boredom, fun, stress, and other leisure times.

So you're probably wondering what is intermittent fasting and  how does it help you lose weight? Well not only is it incredibly effective for helping you lose weight, but its one of the best all natural holistic healing solutions ever!

But before we get into the basics we need to establish a few things. **1.** Fasting is not self-starvation, but volitionally choosing to use calorie restriction, eat less, and have your meals in less frequencies spread out at certain durations of the day. **2.** By intermittent fasting you are restricting food intake for the first half of your day and than later introducing foods at the latter half. You essentially create windows of timeframes you fast under. **3.** Fasting has existed since ancient times and is completely healthy when done under the right supervision. -You can fast for spiritual reasons, political reasons or health conscious reasons.

Fasting is a completely natural phenomenon that aligns itself with our normal physiological functions. In essence fasting is caloric restriction in short, you are restricting the amount of calorie consumption you take in. But what does this do to the human body? *IF* (intermittent fasting) actually has quite a number of positive effects on our bodies and this is backed by science. By intermittent fasting we extend our life span, reverse the aging process, burns excess fat, enhances cardiovascular and brain health, reduce the risk of stroke, high blood pressure, oxidative stress, and improve insulin sensitivity.

Your probably wondering how on earth can fasting have so much benefits and best of all have no side effects like prescription drugs? Did I also mention that it is the most cost affordable solution for everybody on the planet! -You can start completely FREE.

IF is when you don't eat for extended periods of time unlike what we are taught to do by society's cultural norms, which is eating constantly. You create windows of "fasting", meaning you don't eat anywhere between 6- 10 hour intervals, and the frequency of your eating is kept to 1-2 times a day or even eating every other day.

Now if you are starting out its going to be quite the task to readily jump into fasting for 12 hours straight, however, my advise is to build your way up, and note that the first week will probably be your hardest in regards to refraining from eating because your body is just starting to adapt and make the appropriate adjustments.

So start off with 6 hours windows of not eating anything, and keep the frequency at 2 meals per day. Do this for the first week, and when you enter the second week go for 8 hour windows and keep the frequency of eating the same. Once you've hit the 3rd week I suggest either continuing your current regiment or step it up or notch to 10 hour intervals of abstinence and keep the frequency of 1 meal per day.

When you become comfortable you can even take it to the next level and that is eating every other day, meaning you don't eat at all for 24 hours that designated day. Thus, your only consuming food for 4 days out of a 7 day week. This equates to approximately 16 meals within a 30 day calendar month. -Now this is only for those of you who want to follow IF to this extreme, however it's completely fine if you want to do 2 meals per day with 8 hour intervals or 2 meals every other day.

The choice is yours and whichever path you choose you'll notice the weight loss process beginning and you will start to shed those unwanted pounds. By far *IF* is the most effective weight loss strategy that exists because it leverages the body's inherent power and unlocks regenerating, calorie burning, and self-repair mechanisms. Remember no snacking in between any of the periods! -You can have yourself tea or water if you want in between.

I personally eat every other day and keep a 10 hour window and only eat at the frequency of 1 meal, and sometimes 2 meals per day. I didn't do this right away, but in incremental steps as I have previously advised I worked my way up until I was comfortable to live this lifestyle. What did IF do for me?

It had so many health and wellness benefits, I had better mental clarity and sharpness, I was content, mindful and self-aware of my eating habits especially of emotionally triggered eating, I started losing weight rapidly and in a healthy controlled manner, and best of all my muscle definition sculpted to the point where I had almost no body fat. – I must also advise I exercised rigorously and frequently as well. Exercise in conjunction to IF is the ultimate combo and guaranteed way to lose weight and transform your body.

Below I have created an outline for you to follow from beginner, intermediate to advanced in regard to eating schedule. Please feel free to modify the schedule to your individual and unique needs as you see fit. - Nothing is set in stone this is a template. But remember no snacking in between any of the periods!  Later in this book I will cover the best choice food selection, recipes and my personal exercise regiment.

**Beginners IF-**  6 hour intervals & 2 meals per day.


**Beginners IF Stage 2** – 8 hour intervals & 2 meals per day


**Beginners IF Stage 3 –** 8 hour intervals & 1 meal per day


**Intermediate IF –** 10 hour intervals & 1 meal per day


**Intermediate IF stage 2-** 12 hour intervals & 1 meal per day


**Advanced IF –** 1 day intervals (24 hours) & 1 meal every other day




I have just given you a proven and done for you system that has proof of concept and that works! -This has worked wonders for me and many others too. Now its up to you to follow and modify the schedule as you see fit, don't begin until you complete the entire book so you can also incorporate the power foods and some delicious recipes. This is your template to success and all you need to do is follow it and you should start seeing results anywhere between 1-3 weeks! Results will vary depending on the level of fasting you select, foods you choose and if you exercise too. My advice is to work your way up slowly and measure your progress, and than adjust when you feel comfortable. This is as close as we can get to eating like our ancestors and is what I call functional eating. We eat to survive and not for pleasure, however, if you do decide to have your "cheat meals" just ensure it doesn't dramatically alter your schedule or become habitual.

Our forefathers had some incredible insights to life and one of them who is world renowned, Benjamin Franklin, states *"The best of all medicine is resting and fasting".* You heard it straight from the horse's mouth and one of the world's greatest inventors whoever lived and walked the face of planet. He realized something profound that the body inherently possessed its own self-healing, repair mechanisms, and rejuvenating capabilities that don't need to interface with prescription drugs or surgery to attain good health.

This is an incredible truth that one of our forefathers discovered early on, and yet we neglect the power of fasting today although it has been around since ancient times and the dawn of civilization. Every single major religion worldwide regardless of belief, ethnicity, race or creed all incorporate *fasting* as part of spiritual enlightenment. This commonality cannot be disputed we find it among Christians, Hindus, and Buddhist alike whom all engage in periods of fasting at different calendar dates for various reasons. Therefore, it should not come to surprise that fasting has so many benefits that range from anti-aging, healing, enhanced cardiovascular and brain functioning, anti-cancer, anti-inflammation, promotes weight loss, improves insulin sensitivity, and strengthens the immune system.

Ultimately, fasting gives your body a well deserved rest from the foods we are constantly consuming, our bodies can be thought of as sophisticated pieces of machinery and just like any machine requires periods of rest or "cooling off time". – These periods of rest are essential for us to thrive and to function at optimal capacity.

### *How (IF) Boosts Our Health?*

Diabetes – IF lowers insulin the fat storing hormone responsible for excessive weight gain.

Increases human growth hormone – HGH is responsible for increasing muscle mass, increasing life span and just making you look better overall.

Cancer – The number one fueling agent for cancer cells is sugar and by fasting you literally starve cells to death causing "apoptosis", programmed cell death.

Brain health – People have reported to have better mental clarity and sharpness when fasting.

Anti-Aging – You probably thought over indulging in leafy greens and vegetables was the way to go for anti-aging benefits, right? -Well think again! The elixir of life for anti-aging was right under our noses this whole time! That's right fasting promotes remarkable anti-aging benefits, there is a specific molecule called "beta hydroxybutyric" that prevents vascular aging within the body. This is the same molecule that activates under the ketogenic diet when the body switches from burning glucose (sugar) which is a primitive form of utilizing energy to using ketones. -Basically, sugar burning switching to fat burning.

So what does this all mean? The use of beta hydroxybutyric has a chain reaction in the body in specific your DNA, and this change in the body keeps our cells "young" and uncompromised from oxidative stress and free radicals, thus making us immune or less susceptible to chronic degenerative disease states.

High blood pressure – Fasting can reduce high blood pressure due to caloric restriction.

You see fasting has inherent benefits within our bodies, human beings have evolved over the centuries to eat only when necessary. It wasn't until recently we got exposed to excess eating habits, hence, we lived in a time of scarcity and food wasn't always readily available like today because of advanced agriculture. Thus, our bodies adapted and conserved energy from foods we ate for extended periods of times. – It was normal to go days without food back in the day.

You see when you stop eating the hunger hormone called ghrelin gradually decreases in level. Contrary to popular belief you do not become progressively hungrier as time passes! However, the hunger hormone ghrelin secretes itself in waves of intervals and adapts to your unique eating schedule. Now that's a bit of a mind bending paradox, we have all been conditioned to think that if you don't eat you just become progressively and ferociously hungrier.

A controlled experiment using participants had them go for a 30 hour fast. The results were surprising as when ghrelin levels were measured it was observed that ghrelin didn't increase progressively over time, however, but peaked in waves of intervals during the usual eating hours of the participants, and after its peak ghrelin levels decreased and tapered off. – Note that the level of the hunger hormones declined even though participants didn't eat anything!

These periods of hunger the participants experienced were consistent with their usual eating hours at *breakfast, lunch and dinner*. So what does this mean for you? This means when you first start to modify your eating habits to reflect *IF* your feelings of hunger will come and go, and eventually adapt to your new schedule of eating. After a few days your hormones will adapt to your new eating times and you will eventually become less and less hungry.

I can tell you that your first week will be the *hardest* for you to adjust. Remember you spent years developing your habits of eating, but if you stick with the change your body will adapt.

### Mindfulness & Eating

I want to challenge you to really listen to your body the next time your hungry. I want you to practice mindful eating, from each bite, chew slowly, acknowledge the scent, taste and even food's sightful appeal, I want you to savor every moment. By doing this you're really fine tuning your entire appetite and you're no longer mindlessly eating, but self-aware and conscious of every meal you have. Often we find ourselves eating mindlessly, constantly consuming, eating and eating until we are bloated.

Obviously being bloated after our meals is not ideal, and thus the importance of mindful eating. Eating excess causes undue hardship to our bodies, which causes more oxidative stress and requires more work for your body to burn calories.

Humans in the 21$^{st}$ century eat for various reasons apart from survival. We no longer just eat functionally, but we eat because of social reasons, emotional, boredom and for flavor. Interestingly enough when you start practicing mindful eating habits you'll notice you become satisfied quicker than usual and it only takes a few bites of food to do so! You may also notice you don't even need to finish your meal, but a few bites and your body is satisfied, hence the importance of really taking the time to listen to how your body responds to certain foods and act accordingly.

If you need flavor in your diet I suggest incorporating spices or herbs such as salt, oregano, parsley, cayenne pepper, mint and even lemon juice. This way your enhancing taste without all the unwanted calories and your able to satisfy your specific needs.

Lastly, I want to mention relaxing as a strategy while your engage in mindful eating. I know it might sound redundant and obvious, but how many times have you rushed through your meals without giving a second thought to what your eating? Ingesting whatever is in front of you like there's no tomorrow, so you can make it back to work on time from your lunch break.

There are two nervous systems at work your sympathetic nervous system and parasympathetic nervous system. The sympathetic nervous system is responsible for our fight and flight response and anything "stress" related, so imagine if you're in a rush to finish your meal so you can make it back on time for work to please your boss. -You're probably undergoing a certain degree of stress! Thus, you need to cease the moment, plan ahead and take time for yourself to activate the rest and repair nervous system known as the parasympathetic nervous system, which is where resting and healing take place.

### Water & Fiber

Struggling to get full when eating? Why not try incorporating the following simple strategies of increase water and fiber intake? Eat celery or make yourself some celery or vegetable juice which is an excellent source of fiber that can help you reach a state of satiety. Drink more water with your meals, and don't worry it won't dilute your digestive acids contrary to popular belief. Water supports your digestive acids as the more water your intake the more liquid volume you have which makes the entire digestion process much more efficient and fluid for you.

*Salt Deficiency*

Sometimes hunger may arise due to the lack of sodium within our diets. Sodium is required for a plethora of physiological functions from inter-cellular communication to the heart functioning and even needed for optimal nerve transmission.

When insulin levels decrease the more levels of sodium your liver secretes, and hence when you experience bouts of hunger sometimes its just your body's way of telling you its craving some salt. Ergo, when your sodium levels are depleted the body will release insulin to signal you to replenish sodium supply. Thus, the importance of practicing mindful eating so you can try understanding and fine tuning your body's specific needs.

### Insulin, Glycogen, Glucagon & Fasting

When you eat insulin normally goes up and insulin helps you use carbohydrates for energy or stores it as glycogen (deposits of glucose), and when you have too much glycogen stored the incoming carbs your consuming gets converted into fat. Everything we eat spikes insulin, but at different rates, hence, foods that consist of refined carbohydrates massively spike insulin levels when consumed. After about 6 hours after you eat your insulin and blood glucose levels start to diminish, and at this point your pancreas secretes glucagon which has an opposite effect to the hormone insulin.

Insulin is responsible for storing energy, but glucagon releases and pulls energy out of your glycogen and fat storage. Another controlled experiment revealed that injecting animals with insulin increased their food consumption and when animals were injected with glucagon their food consumption greatly decreased.

Now to tie things all together, have you ever wondered why you never get the feeling of satiety for extended periods of time after eating a bowl of cereal or perhaps pasta? You eat these refined carbs and than after maybe 2 hours you get hungry again. Why does this occur? -This is because when you eat refined foods your blood sugar and insulin levels elevate rapidly and cause you to be even more hungry! This happens even after all your meals are processed, and there is excess insulin lingering around. The same goes for when you have your mid-night cravings and munch on some snacks or other refined foods, and than when you wake up in the morning your starving and hungrier than ever before!

Thus when your fasting its actually glucagon that is suppressing your appetite, giving you satiety and burning your stored glycogen and stored fat. There seems to be a common misconception that our brains only run on "glucose", but this is not the case our brain can use *ketones* for fuel by burning fat. As mentioned earlier burning sugar for fuel is a more primitive form of utilizing energy our bodies have evolved and are complex and can use fat burning mechanisms too.

### *Ghrelin & Leptin*

So we know the hormone insulin is tasked with the role of managing blood sugar( glucose) and is responsible for transforming glucose into energy within the intricate and complex systems of our body. But what about the other two hormones known as "ghrelin" and "leptin"? Which are directly responsible for managing our appetite, ghrelin as previously mentioned is the hunger hormone, and leptin is known as our satiety hormone.

People struggling with obesity tend to have these hormones out of whack. Ghrelin runs rampant within the body signaling the body to consume more food, and leptin signaling fails to be received which is responsible for letting you know that you are full or content.

Insulin, ghrelin and leptin work synergistically which ultimately helps us complete a whole myriad of bodily functions and essentially determining if we are hungry or not. So when your hungry be aware that the hormone ghrelin is active within your physiology, and vice-versa when your feeling content the satiety hormone leptin is actively working.

## 5 Common Cravings

There are typically 5 major carvings that humans have which are sweet, salty, sour, spicy and oily (fats). Its no surprise that food manufactures leverage these fundamental cravings within our biology to sell their products to us.

Scientist know if they can trigger our taste buds on our tongue pallet they can elicit our favorable desires for that particular food product. Being aware of these types of cravings is critical to our health and wellness as well because by understanding and fine tuning our body's yearnings we can bring about states of satiety and be content without unhealthily binging on refined foods.

Have you ever tried Keltic sea salt with water? Sometimes it feels so refreshing and rejuvenating as if you have just been recharged, but you'll notice if you continue to drink it the taste will become rancid. Why does this happen? This is due to the bodies need for sodium, hence you start craving salty foods, but once you have replenished your sodium supply anymore salt is excess and unnecessary, ergo the Keltic sea salt drink that was pleasant one moment ago becomes something undesirable. This is simply because our body only needs a certain amount of sodium at a given time, and this principle applies to the other fundamental cravings as well!

Here is the interesting thing, if someone was to put salty chips or perhaps French fries in front of you after you've replenished your sodium supply, and you know this threshold has been reached when the Keltic sea salt drink doesn't taste as appealing to you anymore, guess what?

You probably won't crave the chips or fries because your fundamental salty craving need was met. The human body is an amazing sophisticated piece of biological machinery with many complex intricacies and knows when "enough is enough".

The body knows its daily requirements for essential fats, vitamins, trace minerals and minerals, amino acids, co-factors, and even pro-biotics. The body is an intelligent design and has its own blueprint to function optimally, we just need to provide the right type of raw materials for it to work under its standard operating procedures.

Therefore, whether it's a spicy craving, sour, salty, oily and even sugar craving this could just be our bodies signaling us to replenish supplies of certain elements. You can use this strategies to curb any and all of your food cravings!

However, for sugar I've observed that to curb your sugar cravings you need to do something different. Simply consuming a banana or apple won't necessarily do the trick for cravings of artificial refined sugars as it is more potent. The best way to tackle this problem is intake more protein to curb your sugar cravings, you'll notice the more protein you intake the less you'll crave refined sugars and ultimately your cravings for something sweet will diminish.

By now you probably noticed that your "favorite foods" follow the 5 fundamental cravings all humans have! Is it any wonder why food manufacturers produce their products according to these cravings? If your going into the food industry business you can't go wrong with sweet, salty, sour, spicy and oily foods! – That's why you don't really see bitter or any other type of flavor produced by corporations because they know what your 5 fundamental cravings are and will only design products to exploit them, they know your weak points.

Everything we've come to know and love in the world of food, donuts, hamburgers, pizza, tacos, and other pastries all use either one element or multiple of our 5 fundamental cravings!

### Foods & Inflammation

You've probably faced some form of inflammation in the past from a food you ate which you had an adverse reaction too? The immune system which is heavily housed and can be found within your digestive system is responsible for the defensive response we know as inflammation. The interesting thing about the immune system is that it serves as a duality function meaning the same immune system that heals you from let's say an animal bite wound is the same immune system responsible for heart attacks, joint pain, hives, rashes, redness, headaches and bodily fatigue.

In this section I wanted to talk about common foods that can potentially cause you inflammation and is quite contrary to popular belief. -Foods that the mainstream media endorses as "healthy foods" when can actually cause you a lot of harm.

Let's talk about grains, oats and gluten. I'm sure you have heard about how eating whole grains or oats is good for you by now and its all the buzz in social media and television, but what if I told you that grains can cause you inflammation! You see looking at this from an ecological perspective grains are considered seeds, and nature does not want us eating its seeds. Seeds by design are meant to grow, from seeds sprout apple trees, orange trees, and many other fruit trees.

Since nature doesn't want its seeds eaten as it doesn't serve plants any purpose, thus, these seeds have chemical compounds in them such as gluten to serve as a defensive response to being eaten.

Gluten is just one of many plant defense mechanism that activates when it is consumed. There are other chemical compounds known as phytochemicals called lectin which is associated with digestive issues, arthritis, and autoimmune diseases. Plants have evolved so much that they can produce a form of "birth control" so animals cannot reproduce their offspring, and these birth control chemicals are known as *phytoestrogens*.

This is how advanced plants have become they create defensive phytochemicals when consumed in order to cease the reproduction of offspring down the line, so their seeds cannot be eaten. So you probably think well if I eat gluten free oats, brownies, pizza, etc your going to be alright?- Think again, as mentioned earlier plants have a whole range of phytochemicals that they use in response to being eaten, and gluten is just one of the many phytochemicals.

But I thought oats were healthy? – Yes, they do have healthy nutritional components to them such as fiber, healthy oils, vitamin E, and protein. But you can think of this as a double edged sword, and although it has many health benefits there is potential risks for inflammation.

The best way to figure out if oats or grains effect you is to eat them and observe what happens! Plant seeds want to preserve their survival so they can grow and hence use defensive response chemicals to punish animals or humans to decide to eat them.

***Socially Engineered To Constantly Eat – Corporations
Vested Interest***

In my introduction I briefly touched on how animals in
the wild don't eat out of boredom, but out of necessity
to survive. I painted you the example of the content lion
whom we consider king of the jungle and a ferocious
beast. However, interestingly enough when even these
majestic creatures are content, they do no hunt for prey
to eat.

So who came up with this whole notion to constantly be
eating at almost every part of our day? We are
bombarded constantly with commercials from
McDonalds, KFC, Burger King, etc and the motive
behind these marketing tactics is to take your money!
You see corporations behind all the fast food chains and
the entire food empire per se have their own vested
interests to sell to you and it is certainly not for your
benefit. They have ulterior motives and could careless
about your health and wellness!

I want you to think critically who designed this
framework of eating breakfast, lunch and dinner, and of

course "snacking" in between with more junk food? Breakfast, lunch and dinner have been commercialized so much to condition us that we don't even question it! -Its just a normal part of life going through the drive-thru of McDonalds to get our fix. Corporations are the most anti-human entities on the planet, they could careless about your health and wellness. Did you know fast food franchises and as a matter of fact the entire food empire hire food scientists to do their "dirty work"? – What do I mean by this?

Well, you see food scientist are hired to design and manufacture foods that are addictive to you and me. That's right I said addictive, the same kind of addiction drug addicts have is essentially the same results they try to emulate from us too, and is it any coincidence that the primary go to ingredient for almost all food additives is some form of sugar!

That's right I said sugar! I am not talking about the kind of sugar our body uses for fuel (glucose) although excess amounts can be harmful as previously discussed, however, I am specifically talking about refined and processed sugar that food manufactures incorporate into all their products. There are actually different types of sugars and corporations have become sneaky and have concealed the generally known term of sugar by using other forms, substitutes or sweeteners.

We need to become proficient label deck readers in order to understand the kinds of foods we are eating. But  a general rule of thumb to keep you safe is anything found at the supermarket that can be bought in a cardboard box and has an extended shelf-life should be considered harmful to your health.

Now let's go over the different forms of sugar and artificial sweeteners that you may not be able to easily recognize at first glance.

### *6 Types of Sugars to Lookout For*

**Dextrose**

**Fructose**

**Sucrose**

**Maltose**

**Lactose**

**Galactose**

## *Artificial Sweeteners to Lookout For*

Saccharin

Aspartame

Corn Syrup

Advantame

Neotame

Stevia

Acesulfame

## Substitute For Sugars to Lookout for

**Molasses**

**Honey**

**Xylitol**

**Brown rice syrup**

**Coconut palm sugar**

**Date sugar**

**Maple Syrup**

**Agave Syrup**

**Brown rice Syrup**

**Coconut Palm Sugar**

We need to become aware of the many hidden forms of sugar food manufacturing corporations sneak into our foods. Hence, the importance of becoming a proficient ingredient deck label reader!

A statistic revealed that the average American eats excess amounts of 200,000 lbs of sugar every single year! The fact is we only need a table spoon of sugar (natural) within our blood stream at any given point in time. Sugar can be a dangerous substance and has volatile characteristics and simply put it can make things explode literally!

You see because sugar can be explosive our bodies have evolved to develop complex mechanisms and procedures to store sugar efficiently.  Due to the explosive nature of sugar the hormones insulin facilitates the transferring of excess sugar to fat, and hence why we see refined sugar being the primary cause of weight gain in North America.

### *Sugar Addiction*

Sugar addiction is a real thing as strange as it may sound people have addictions to sugar! Corporations have exploited this drive we all posses inherently and the craving for something sweet which elicits feelings of euphoria. Corporations go to the extreme in order to get us hooked they actually do lab experiments on people by having them enter the *MRI* while eating a particular food that can be a chocolate bar, chips, etc and what this does is it reveals brain activity through the MRI, and scientist use this information to insidiously craft food products.

Our brains light up at certain regions which corresponds to the stimulus consumed (food) and scientist take a close look at the regions that have been stimulated and design their food products accordingly.

You'd probably be surprised to know that usually all these mega food franchises like McDonald's, Harveys, Subway, Burger King, Dunkin' Donuts and many more companies share the same supplier that provides them carefully crafted and specifically designed food products that have addictive properties. Some sort of food manufacturing plant that has food-scientist working for them to create the "secrete" or ideal recipes that make these companies their fortune. – Sounds like something out of science fiction, right? – But the sad truth is this is far from fiction and is the reality we live in.

There was a scientific study   conducted by the University of Bordeaux in France by *Dr. Serge Ahmed* who was using rats in a controlled experiment, and this experiment entailed sugar and cocaine as the stimulus. Both researchers and Dr. Serge were surprised at the outcome of this experiment because the rats were given both cocaine and sugar and they wanted to know which was the preferred stimulus. To their shock the rats actually choose sugar over cocaine! -That's right they choose refined sugar over the notorious drug *cocaine.*

The study revealed the addictive powers of sugar and why it's a substance to be leery of and something to be avoided. This explains a lot actually if you really come to think about it? We see in this modern day people who cannot control their eating habits or should I say binge eating habits when it comes to  refined sugar. I have a challenge for you or perhaps this is something you can be made aware of if you think back. Have you ever tried an Oreo cookie, chips maybe Doritos or your favorite pack of donuts? – Can you honestly tell me that you've only stopped at eating one? Truthfully, you most likely demolished the whole box!

The simple fact is you couldn't control yourself to the addictive appeal of sugar! " It just taste so darn good", sweet yet addictive and harmful to your well being, eliciting feelings of bliss and euphoria, and let's not forget responsible for the degeneration of health and the catalyst to many chronic degenerative diseases when you have constant exposure to it over time.

The issue here is humans have mastered the craft of manipulating almost anything into specific concentrations, for instance, heroin comes from poppy seeds, cocaine from coco plants, and alcohol from grains. In their natural forms these plant components are quite harmless, however when precisely extracted into concentrations is where the trouble arises. These are naturally occurring substances we get from our planet, but through devious manipulation techniques and procedures these pristine substances produce addictive compounds!

Food manufacturing corporations and scientist probably have a laugh saying " I dare you to try just one", and I'm sure this is probably a slogan that a food company probably used in their marketing camping  at some point in time, however, they know deep down inside they are manipulating our biology and exploiting our built in drives to create habitual forming products that are engineered to be simply irresistible!

The industrialization and advance agriculture of our society is wherein lies the problem, when we refine these substances in their most concentrated form to get you hooked, and is where the addiction and misery of many people over the century was born.

## Historical Corporate Use of Addictive Substances

Coca-Cola arguably the world's most successful soft drink brand that came into existence in the late 19<sup>th</sup> century has used questionable substances in the past that gave "coke" its addictive quality. Even this big brand name has some skeletons in the closet. Did you know in the early 1900s Coca-Cola actually had trace amounts of cocaine in it?! Yes, this is not a myth, but the truth is Coca-Cola used cocaine in specific concentrations in varying amounts which most likely gave "coke" its addictive hook. It must be noted that cocaine was *legal* at the time during the periods of *1886 – 1929* and was used for medicinal purposes, and cocaine is still used today for medical purposes.

But eventually the government regulatory bodies caught up and prohibited the use of cocaine publicly, especially in food. Thus, cocaine was outlawed and Coca-Cola had to find a new addictive ingredient and they turned to refined ***sugar*** and ***caffeine*** which is still used till this day.

I don't think I have to go into details of why caffeine is addictive as well I'm pretty sure you know by now this substance also contains habitual forming addictive properties and is used by all fast food restaurant chains worldwide when they're serving you your "morning fix".

*SLIP*

Have you heard of the term SLIP? This is terminology used by food scientist and describes the phenomenon of the rate at which food slips down your throat. Fast food manufactures are privy to this information and exploit it because they know our human biology, and the faster food slips down our throat the more we will potentially eat. Why is this?

When we eat normally we chew our foods into a mushy paste before swallowing and this also prepares our digestive enzymes and other biochemical processes within our body, and food manufactures know that this requires a lot of energy, thus they try to trick our bodies by expediting the journey of food and making it travel down our digestive system faster so that way we can continue to eat more! -They understand that the more we chew foods, specifically foods that are natural (whole foods) the more work is required for our bodies to utilize energy, and thus the less food we will eat.

Ergo, refining foods is to their advantage as they have been stripped bare and have little to know fiber or nutrition, hence why we can consume loads of refined foods in a single sitting versus eating whole foods which fill us up much faster with much less.

As you can see the people, or should I say corporations behind all the big food brands that you crave have figured us all out. By deconstructing our basic and fundamental human biology and exploiting our biochemistry to push their irresistible products to us so they can make a fortune. They are literally pushing our buttons and manipulating us through flavor and other appealing features. You may argue well, we have free choice or free moral agency to do whatever we choose; however, you must understand that there is a toxic miasma present and food manufactures are exploiting our very biology in order to control us. When is the last time you had only one Oreo cookie or ate one piece of chip from your favorite junk food brand? -The answer is most likely never! This is because its almost as if we don't have a choice, but to eat their food via the manipulation of our senses.

Therefore, it is so important to be aware and follow my strategies in order to be liberated from this *food empire's* tyranny. We need to understand intermittent fasting, mindful eating, and the power of whole foods which I will discuss later in this book, and the consequences of eating "Frankenstein foods". These substances used in our modern day food supply are habit forming, and thus keep us coming back for more and more with dire consequences to our health that corporations could care less about!

Even from the way foods are packaged, designed and boxed have all been scientifically proven to captivate us and thus make us purchase their product. Next time you go to McDonalds I want you to observe how the packaging is, and soon you'll notice similarities to how opening up that *big mac* that has been wrapped up for you is likened to opening Christmas gifts!

What do I mean by this? Food manufactures have studied the psychology behind us, what makes us tick, what makes us happy, and ultimately why we desire things. They know the psychology behind our buying habits so much that they even understand emulating "gift-wrap" for Christmas creates a sense of excitement and joy sub-consciously when we are unwrapping our foods from the wrapper. They know by subtly exploiting our sub-conscious drives as well they can enhance our experience when we participate in their products. Hence the importance of being aware of these things and reverse hacking the exploits they have put us under.

## Intermittent Fasting – The Best Anti- Aging Strategy

Earlier int this book I mentioned anti-aging is one of the many benefits of IF. If we break IF down at its most fundamental level we are essentially looking at "caloric restriction", which simply put is restricting the calories you consume. Besides who do you think came up with the notion of constantly eating throughout the day? – I can give you a hint its starts with a "*c*" and I am sure you guessed by now, if you guessed corporations your absolutely right! Of course, corporations want you eating more its in their vested interest that you are eating their products throughout the day. They want you to buy more and more and could care less about you as an individual, however they're more concerned with making money.

This is a vicious cycle if you look at it from the outside, imagine this, you eat poorly and as a result you have poor health and you have to go to the doctors for medical intervention for whatever disease you're stuck with because of your poor food choices. The result is both physical and financial misery, and what a terrible way to live life! – But by the end of this book I hope you will break this vicious cycle!

Caloric restriction is not complicated at all! The less you eat the less load or less work is required from your body. The more work our bodies are subject too the faster we age, and thus the higher chance of susceptibility to chronic diseases. The more metabolic work our body is involved with the shorter our lifespan will be, and a controlled study conducted with lab animals proves this point. There were two groups of mice group *A* and group *B,* group A was given the standard diet, but group B was denied food and put under caloric restriction. In short group B lived significantly longer than their counterparts and lived healthier!

Group A's lifespan was cut much shorter and they seemed to acquire chronic diseases much more easily. Case in point the power of caloric restriction for anti-aging and longevity.

I hear misinformation left, right and centre and one time on T.V I heard a supposed fitness "expert" claiming that we should raise our metabolism. First off, I want to tell you this is a terrible idea and raising your metabolism will do nothing good for you health-wise. We should have   our metabolic rate strong, stable and slow, not fast. Our metabolism can be defined as the sum total of all our bodily chemical reactions, both chemicals that build up our body and break down our body.

Did you know animals that live shorter lives have faster metabolisms? – And animals that live long have slow and steady metabolisms. You see the more energy the body spends on digestion, absorption, and processing foods the less energy it will have to spend on anti-aging, building muscle, and both growth and repair functions. As you can see eating more is a disservice to our bodies and causes a lot more harm than good, on top of that interestingly enough when our bodies run low on energy this is when the emergency response system kicks in and we run into some serious problems.

The point is you don't want to raise your metabolism; however, you want to re-allocate where energy is spent within your metabolism and balance things out that is the key. It doesn't matter if your only eating healthy too whether its salad, lean meat, etc this is all still considered work for the body! Digestion, absorption, allocating energy and expelling waste all requires your body to work.

Just like any machine the body needs rest too. So, what happens if you don't give your body the deserved rest it requires? Remember earlier I mentioned if your body runs low on energy meaning your constantly eating not giving it any rest, then this is when the emergency response kicks in. Its sort of like having to many applications working on your computer and the system is overwhelmed and freezes, and than your forced to go into "safe mode" , and in this mode you can only use your computer at its most basic functions and features. In this same way when you're constantly eating and forcing your body to work **24/7 365** days year round your body will not perform at its optimal potential.

Just like how you need to go on vacation from work every now and than, your body also needs to go on "holiday" from eating too. You see when you take a break from food your body can now use its precious resources on things like repair, healing, strengthening, growth and anti-aging because energy can be redistributed into these avenues. – The whole digestion process is a lot of work. Do you ever get sleepy after a big meal? Well that's because digestion is extremely taxing on the body.

Now you can see why eating 5-6 meals a day is a very bad idea and so is messing with your metabolism. Some people and even dietitians have this misinformed concept that eating food all day like how cows graze on grass all day is good for you, but they are sadly mistaken. – **Cows have four stomachs, while humans only have one!**

### Diabetes & Fasting

Earlier in this chapter I touched briefly and discussed the hormone insulin and its relation to glycogen and glucagon. I want to elaborate further on the role of insulin and its connection to diabetes, and also how fasting can drastically improve and even reverse this chronic condition.

I mentioned when you eat anything insulin is up-regulated meaning its actively working, and is responsible to tell cells when to divide, grow and manage blood sugar levels. Now imagine if your constantly eating which is the primary stimulus for insulin secretion, the body eventually becomes numb to insulin due to over exposure, and hence you get something called insulin sensitivity which is the hallmark of type 2 diabetes.

Cells become resistant and stop listening. This is when a plethora of problems arise; heart, blood pressure, brain, auto-immune disease, and inflammation all stem from insulin resistance and doctors have coined this fancy term as metabolic syndrome which basically means your whole body is out of whack or messed up.

Fasting just a few days can help revitalize your body's response to insulin. Having insulin resistants only prolongs your overweight problem as you'll start to store more fat in your cells as oppose to burn them. The thing is although your body becomes unresponsive to insulin in regard to cell feeding, however, the body will continue storing fat continuously, and this is why we see a lot of the times generally speaking people with diabetes tend to have weight issues.

Hence, why the importance of fasting cannot be understated. As soon as you start to fast you will see that metabolic syndrome symptoms start to disappear and eventually reverse. Your diabetes won't heal overnight but will take time and with the right nutritional protocol alongside with IF you will be able to regain your health.

*Exercise & Intermittent Fasting*

Whether your body building or just trying to get in shape IF enhances your body capacity to build muscle! When you start to fast between 1-2 days between workout periods genes called sirtuins activate, which are linked anti-aging and muscle building.

I'm sure you heard about how resting is as important as weight lifting when it comes to gaining muscle, and much is the same with the principle of fasting. Your body needs rest from the constant processing of food and the many biochemical procedures required, and by doing so the body can redistribute energy to other departments such as body building, fat burning, repair and growth.

### Not All Calories Are Made Equal

You hear a lot of dietitian and even doctors talk about calories, but never really make the distinction between empty calories and dense calories full of nutrition. This is a big disservice to the general public as this misleads the masses to assume that all calories are equal which is not the case. Not all calories are made equal!

Refined and processed foods contain mostly empty calories, remember these foods have been stripped of their nutrients, minerals and vitamins perhaps at best they have some sort of additive like fiber to enhance the product, but nonetheless overall its still junk food. Whole foods on the other hand are calorie dense packed with essential nutrients, fats, fiber and other trace minerals that your body requires to function optimally.

This is a distinction that you must be made aware of because many people are mislead to believe eating calories from a baked pizza is the same as calories from a healthy salad bowl. – Calories are not all the same, thus be cognizant of the type of calorie your eating, especially if your one to measure your daily caloric intake.

### *Don't Use Willpower To Fast*

I'm a firm believer in willpower when it comes to pursuing your dreams, ambition and fulfilling your goals in life. However, when it comes to built in hard-wired human drives I am not so much a big advocate when it comes to fasting and consuming foods. Now this might sound puzzling or quite paradoxical because your thinking you need to have a certain measure of willpower to abstain from junk foods, and your probably right to a certain degree you do need a resolve and determination to refrain from unhealthy foods.

But, I am a firm believer in promoting satiety over willpower, and by this we are hacking into our base internal drives at the most fundamental and instinctive levels. Think about it we are up against corporations who have been exploiting our built in drives for over centuries now, and thus it would make sense for us to fight back by "flipping the script" and reverse engineering what they've done to us.

How do we do this? Consume a diet rich in whole foods, protein, coconut oils, meats and healthy fats! – I will go into more details about this later in the book, but that is basically the gist of it. Finding ways to curb our cravings for refined foods by replacing them with foods that can meet our built in drives.

Willpower alone is useless, and I wouldn't recommend solely relying on willpower for fasting. As mentioned before your first week of IF will probably be your hardest, but once you have broken into it you will start to get the hang of it and understand your body in a more deeper and intimate way. You'll be able to start fine tuning your needs and truly understand hunger.

A lot of the times when we eat we are not actually hungry but have been programmed by society to eat. You'll notice when you start fasting there is a distinct difference between psychological eating and physiological eating. When you eat psychologically its due to social conditioning and not the true need to eat, but when you eat physiologically its for functionality and the need to survive like the animals in the wild.

Remember I am not asking you to starve yourself, but to take extended periods of times or windows and fast. Don't jump into it cold turkey but follow my instructions and incrementally build your way up to your comfort level. The truth is everybody should fast as a health protocol and benefit, not enough of us do and suffer from many health problems consequently. Once you've become accustom to IF you'll realize that your "old hunger" becomes more of a mental sensation than a physical need.

I don't believe in using willpower to control in our built in drives, however, we need to learn how to manage and guide our cravings by using nutritional strategies.

## Things To Consider

Many diets propose a one size fits all method and this is inherently wrong and contains many erroneous principles behind it. We know every individual is unique and will need a specialized approach and diet plan designed for their specific needs. Earlier I discussed the 5 fundamental cravings and each person has their own preferred desirable taste, every individual will like one taste appeal over the other.

However, when it comes to fasting everyone benefits from it regardless of age. But, the only exception is the intensity of the fast as each person is equipped to handle IF at different levels as we are all unique and have different physiological needs and capacities.

Have you ever watched the show "Biggest Loser", I'm sure you've heard of this program on T.V before? Contestants who are obese go on the show and take on a challenge to lose weight within a certain set period of time. A big component not publicized enough apart from diet modifications like the ketogenic or low carb diet, - fasting is at the forefront and aids participants in losing large amounts of weight. Simply put they restrict calories and utilize IF.

But, interestingly enough you never really hear from the participants again after their showtime run finishes. On other reality shows there is usually some sort of "reunion" type of theme, but in this case, we don't really see that. One should also note that participants do sign a non disclosure agreement which make sense why we don't really hear much from them.

Now what point am I trying to get across? Well, did you know a good amount of these contestants lose weight successfully, but after a short period of time gain it all back!

To understand this, we must dig deeper and understand what happens to us when we eat. So, we know when we eat insulin is secreted in varying amounts, and sugar and fat are stored in the liver. But when to much incoming sugar appears your body starts to convert and store fat in excess amounts.

There is this flawed notion and I'm pretty sure you've heard this popular phrase "calories in and calories out", which is very flawed. As explained earlier not all calories are made equal and depending on various factors including biochemistry and what type of calorie you consume will dictate if it is stored or burned. So, what happens when you have insulin insensitivity? Does your body burn fat as effectively according to the calorie in calorie out model? Absolutely not, because without insulin delegating storing and fat burning you will not be able to access the fat burning mechanisms due to the lack of responsiveness of insulin, hence the importance of "re-sensitizing" your insulin hormone through IF.

This is why we see so many contestants fail in the long run because they are simply following a flawed system and model that simply does not work. Neglecting the whole picture and ignoring the crucial master hormone insulin does people a disservice, and now we can see why these contestants gain back all their weight.

There is this popular myth out there about if you fast your going to "burn muscle", and I can tell you this is false. Studies confirm this that your protein is preserved and stays intact as oppose to being burned as many mistakenly think. Rest assure IF will not burn lean muscle, however it is possible you may not build as fast or become as "big" due to the lack of protein intake. But, overall IF will enhance muscle building and repair processes.

## Different Forms of Fasting

There are different types or forms of fasting that you can try. Ideally the cessation of all food consumption is the best type of fast, but if you want when starting out you can try the following types of fasts to get you familiar with the process. Than you can slowly work your way up to higher level fasts mentioned in the book in incremental steps.

Types of Fast:

*Fruit Juice fast*

*Vegetable juice fast*

*Smoothie fast*

*Water fasts*

***Why Intermittent Fasting is a Foolproof Strategy***

The ultimate detox, cleanse and universally accessible weight loss method is intermittent fasting! Anybody can do it! People from all ages, whether your male or female it doesn't matter. There is absolutely no reason why you cannot start IF today! Its completely free so what is your excuse?

Think about it with intermittent fasting you don't have to shop, clean or even meal prep anything! Whether your vegan, don't eat meat, have nut allergies, don't have money or travel the bottom line is you can still fast!

Advantages of Intermittent Fasting:

-Simple

-Free

-Accessible

-Healthy

- Convenient

-Flexible

-Start anytime

- No restrictions

-Safe (Preferably under medical supervision)

- Allows body to rest

- Enables growth, repair and regenerative capacities

- Helps with muscle preservation and definition

- Cleanses & detox Body

- Restores balance

- Longevity & increased life span

- Anti-aging benefits

Its incredible that such a simple yet profound technique that has been known since ancient times can be used to improve your health from a holistic standpoint. Remember our bodies are like machines and thus we need to take special care of this sophisticated piece of machinery we have been blessed with and you can start improving your health and losing weight simply by fasting!

### *Bariatric Surgery - Gastric Sleeve & Gastric By-Pass*

If you have ever considered getting a gastric sleeve done which is also known as a "bariatric surgery" I want to give you the facts and my take on surgery for weight loss. Surgery for weight loss can be effective but is NOT something I recommend to anyone! I don't really see it as a health promoting effort nor something long term without complications.

So, what exactly is a gastric sleeve? Well doctors literally cut up your stomach and resize it to 15% of its original size and use medical grade staples to close the incisions. A gastric by-pass which is also a medical procedure is when a surgeon divides your stomach into smaller upper pouches which is rearranged to connect to your small intestine. – There are many variations of this medical procedure.

Now I am just appalled that this is even a remotely available option here in the 21$^{st}$ century, nothing can be more barbaric than having someone go inside your body, cut, solder, and rearrange your organs in order to help you lose weight. Is it just me that thinks that this is a little insane? – Of course, the procedure works effectively, but what they don't tell you is the long term complications that come with it!

In theory it sounds good that by reducing the size of your stomach you also thereby decrease appetite and your capacity to eat. But let's look at some of the complications and risks associated with bariatric surgery that aren't highlighted or nearly emphasized enough!

*Complications & Risks to Bariatric Surgery:*

- *Bowel* obstructions
- *Loss of urinary control*
- *Puking & Vomiting*
- *Bleeding*
- *Gall bladder rupture*
- *Fatigue*
- *Ulcers*
- *Depression from other side effects*
- *Nausea*
- *Painful digestion*
- *Inability to control defecating*
- *-Chronic pain*
- *Death*

These are only a small list of complications and side effects that you will experience after surgery, and there are many more. You can expect frequent visits to the hospital due to all the complications, but what do you expect you allowed a surgeon to go inside of you and literally butcher your organs!

I wrote this book to save you from going down this road and let you know that there are other alternatives that are much safer, effective and healthier than going in for surgery. Please, I admonish you and even beg you to listen to my advice as you will have regret going down the path of weight loss surgery. I have met many people who have had this procedure done and they all regret it! -It really is a short lived experience, and while you may rapidly lose weight initially, but you will be living with long term health complications that will seriously affect your quality of life.

Not only is it a physical burden but also a financial one too. The surgery itself is quite expensive, and you may get lucky enough to have insurance cover it, but I can tell you that there will be even bigger expenses down the road due to the complications that the surgery brings. Its not natural for the body to be cut open and have its organs removed, resized or even rearranged.

There is this propaganda being fed to the masses and that its in your genes to be "fat" or overweight. Who do you think this serves? Definitely not you, but the agenda of corporations, and you can see an almost symbiotic relationship with food corporations producing foods that cause diseases including obesity, and than hospitals having to treat you for your ailments. It's a vicious cycle and extremely profitable business model. Its almost as if food manufactures and the modern medical system are in collusion together!

This so anti-human on so many levels. What benefit does this really serve you except a series of unfortunate events that will unfold due to you putting your trust in the medical model. Remember your battle is with addictive and habitual forming foods that use substances that exploit our built in drives. Genes are secondary to lifestyle and environmental influences, meaning your genes turn on and off like lights and are secondary to the decisions you make and what you expose yourself too.

Although genes contain the blueprint and play an integral role in determining certain physical attributes or the expression of them, however, genes alone don't cause obesity! Imagine a plane crash, do we blame gravity for this? Certainly not, although gravity is fundamental and so are genes, but the direct cause and effect cannot originate from gravity alone. But, the events preceding the plane crash, such as human error, mechanical issues, terrorism or even weather. Do you understand now why genes are secondary?

The human body is an intelligent design and is so sophisticated that it knows what it needs. Posses renewing, regenerating capabilities, and self-healing mechanisms that are inherently found within everyone's body! This is a divine gift that everyone posses and has access too. The key is to learn how to leverage this healing system, and that is through proper nutrition, exercise and fasting!

Any doctor telling you to go the route of bariatric surgery needs to be fired! – And held accountable. Without even touching on other alternative health strategies that work, and to solely have you go down this path for their financial gain is a crime to humanity. So why isn't fasting endorsed by our medical professionals that we hold on a pedestal?

*Because there is no money!* That's right, no financial gain!  What would it profit the medical system to endorse fasting? They wouldn't be able to make money off telling you a strategy that is completely free, non-invasive, safe, and even more effective than weight loss surgery. This is the world we are living in and that's why its incredibly important to become self-aware. The purpose of this entire book is to give you the truth and nothing but the truth, and of course holistic strategies you can use for weight loss.

Fasting has proven time and time again that it is the ultimate weight loss strategy that exists from even ancient times. Doctors know this but seem to only promote their own agenda.

Thus, if you have ever considered bariatric surgery, please take time to reconsider and really analyze the facts, and weigh the risks versus outcome. Its not worth doing as its really a short cut and all short cuts come with immense repercussions.

You will lose weight through IF, but you just need to take action, stick with the program, and trust the process.

**Summary of Intermittent Fasting**


You've reached the end of this chapter and I would like to give you a small recap of what you learnt. IF has existed since ancient times and has been observed to elicit immense health benefits ranging from weight loss, repair and growth, regeneration and healing. Below are terms I would like to clarify in case you may have gotten confused, and note I provide you a glossary at the end of the book for definitions.


*Intermittent fasting* – Periodic fasting at any given period of time. 8 hour, 6 hour , 12 hour or even 24 hour windows before you eat.


*Calories restriction – Eating less food or consuming less calories by eating less food.*


*Fasting – Refraining from consuming food.*


The distinction between hunger for functional eating and hunger for habitual or psychosocial eating must be known. You must be aware of the mind and body disconnect because only than you can truly understand if you are truly hungry or not.

Hence, the importance of mindful eating and becoming aware, find tuning your body's physiological needs versus psychological wants. Your mind can be your greatest ally or foe depending on how you condition it! Meaning if you let your mind take control and allow it to dictate your eating behavior based on craving substances that exploit our built in drives than you will surely lose the battle.

But if you focus and listen to what your body is telling you and practice functional eating like animals in the wild you will come on top every time. Remember there are various hormones at play when eating and fasting, but the three major hormones at the forefront are insulin, ghrelin and leptin.

Ghrelin is responsible for feeling of hunger and is released in waves of intervals and does not progressively build up contrary to popular belief. Leptin is responsible for satiety and leveraging this hormone is essential to achieve states of contentment. Insulin is considered a master hormone of sorts and is responsible for delegating sugar and fat burning and storage, and as well as many more functions.

Like insulin resistance, leptin resistance is a phenomenon that occurs within people who struggle with excess weight. Leptin tells you to stop eating, but we see some people are unresponsive to leptin and thus don't get the "I'm satisfied" signal and continue to consume more food than required. Thus, not only does IF re-sensitizes your response to insulin, but also re-sensitizes your response to leptin, thereby helping you feel satisfied when you eat again.

You can think of it as a full body reset just like how you reset your computer when multiple browsers are open causing you to lag.

Once you're in a state of fasting your body now can focus and allocate its precious resources to healing, growth and repair mechanisms, and no longer divert energy to processing foods via digestion. Basically, your body gets to do some much needed maintenance or "spring cleaning" when you fast.

The incredible benefits of IF cannot be emphasized enough, through fasting you can relief auto-immune diseases temporarily, reduce seizures, lowers cholesterol, revitalizes skin, sharpens your alertness and much, much more!

***Warnings to Consider:***

Before starting any new regiments please consult your doctor or licensed health care professional and see if there may be any risks or health complications associated with IF due to your current circumstances.

Also, if you are struggling with high levels of insulin low blood sugar levels may cause you migraines, therefore consult your doctor and ask how you can incorporate a modified IF to your lifestyle.

## Chapter 2: Chronic Degenerative Diseases & Unhealthy Living

What if diseases were due to nutritional deficiencies and the exposure to toxins? – This is exactly what constitutes all chronic disease states and I will cover this subject matter in more in depth details in the following.

By the end of this book I want you to become your own authoritative figure and make your own informed decisions. Be skeptical always and think critically especially when watching mainstream media.

This chapter will be dedicated to chronic degenerative diseases states and its correlation to a sedentary lifestyle or unhealthy living. I figured I might as well dedicate a whole chapter to this subject matter, so you can grasp the entire picture of health and wellness and have a multifaceted understanding and not a one dimensional concept.

The first thing we need to understand is that everything occurs at the level of a cell. What is a cell? A cell is what composes our organs, tissues, bones and many other bodily appendages. There are many intricate components to a cell or you can think of them as sub-departments that have their own independent functions. I won't go into details in regards to *cell organelles* as this is not a science text book, but I just want you to grasp the fundamental concept of a cell.

In today's modern world we are bombarded with new prescription drugs almost every other month. Essentially poisons that manipulate our body's biochemistry to suppress inflammation, inhibit activity, or forcefully produce results artificially. The average person doesn't realize that when your interfacing with pharmaceutical drugs to treat our chronic diseases we are playing with fire!

Now I am not saying we don't ever need drugs, I'm not being overly optimistic, however, there is a time and a place for medical intervention through drugs. But, has your doctor ever recommended taking nutrition or even fasting as a viable option to restore your health? Probably not because he doesn't get paid to endorse these kinds of solutions by drug manufactures, and doctors treat things at the level of symptomologies as oppose to targeting the underlying root problems holistically.

This is what has become of our western medical model, prescription drugs and invasive procedures that are more or less a band-aid style approach to treating sickness. How is it that our society becomes sicker and sicker with these current standards of treatments? -The answer is simple these treatments do not work long term but alleviate short term symptoms by ignoring the underlying root casual level.

Every bodily breakdown happens at the level of a cell. Nutrition plays a crucial role to the integrity of our health and wellness. Basically, all chronic degenerative disease states 1. Occur at the level of a cell. 2. Diseases are the lack of nutritional deficiencies and exposure to toxins. Perhaps the premature death of many people here in the industrialized world boils down to the starvation of essential nutrients?

You see as I mentioned before prescription drugs have a time and place for usage, and if we are using them to alleviate discomfort in the short term I'm completely fine with that and even recommend it. However, when doctors start prescribing patients prescription drugs long term as viable option for treatment, then I put my foot down and cannot stand for this. Prescription drugs are one of the leading causes of death in America, and your doctor is certainly not helping the cause! You see all you do is mask symptoms with drugs without ever tackling the root problem.

Drugs only poison the body to cover symptoms and essentially creating a falsehood of "good health", and we think this is ok?

So ok by now you understand the determinantal effects of prescription drugs, but can nutrition and fasting really be used as medicine to treat chronic diseases? Yes! Absolutely, we see this time and time again people reversing their diseases with the right nutritional protocol and elimination of food toxicity.

I mentioned earlier in the last chapter how the body is an amazing piece of sophisticated machinery that only requires the right raw materials to function optimally. Still don't believe me that everyone has an intelligent self-healing system that is inherent within our body? The next time you cut your finger observe and see what happens, and you will see the marvelous intelligence and self-repair mechanism of your body at work. What happens when you cut yourself? You bleed yes, but what happens after without you even thinking or giving a command?

Your body starts to repair itself on its own! -You didn't even need to think it! Platelets come to the cover and patch up the wound in a matter of seconds, and the healing process begins almost instantly. Now do you see how your body is a healing system capable of taking care of itself as long as the right conditions are met.

Now lets discuss nutrition. You need to understand the fundamentals of nutrition in order to use it correctly. The following are the fundamentals of nutrition.

### Fundamental Nutritional Building Blocks

-Protein – best sources whey powder, bone soup & eggs.

-Fats – Essential fatty acids, salmon, Herring, Sardines, Halibut.

- Carbs – Leafy green vegetables, cabbage, Romanian salad, carrots, cucumbers, and you can also add olive or coconut oils as dressing.

-Water - Filtered Water. Our bodies are electrical system and use electrical currents when minerals and water are combined in conjunction.

-Vitamins 2 types: Fat soluble & Water soluble.

Fat soluble = Vitamin D, A, E, K.

Water soluble = B Vitamin complex & Vitamin C.

-Minerals – Zinc, Silica, copper, magnesium, chromium, and vanadium.

- Trace minerals & nutrients – selenium, NAC.

-Probiotics – Lactobacillus acidophilus, Bifidobacterium bifidum.

All the above listed nutrition constitutes your fundamental building blocks for health and wellness.

## *Inflammation*

We all have had some sort of inflammation at some point or the other in our life. We take medication in order to alleviate inflammation and the inconvenience it brings to us, and although relieving symptoms that irritate us in the short term is ok for comfort, however its when we do this in the long term without addressing the root problem.

So what is inflammation? First of all we need to understand why inflammation occurs in the first place! Inflammation is apart of our immune system and is our body's defensive response to something that triggers our system. That's right inflammation is our body's way of protecting itself from an intruder, thus instead of knocking down the immune system as solution we need to figure out what is causing the immune system to be triggered.

That would be the most logical move according to deductive reasoning, thus, we need to find out why our body is responding in a defensive fashion and what exactly is the catalyst to this trigger. Therefore, anytime you have inflammation you need to think what is causing this to happen? – Long term use of immune system suppression through drugs can literally shut down your immune response for other essential things, for instance imagine you're a long term user of a prescription drug that suppresses inflammation causing pain for arthritis, and you get into a car accident or you have a nasty slip and fall. Your recovery from the accident will be almost non-existent and you could potentially die easier because your immune system has been suppressed for so long.

Do you see the dangers for long term use of immune suppressing drugs? -And I should say any prescription drug for that matter. There are really only three ways your immune system can be activated and that's through your respiratory tract, digestive tract and skin contact. In other words, breathing, eating and direct skin contact are really the only possible entry points where your body mounts a defensive response which means inflammation!

For most people its usually eating! Thus, any sort of immune response associated with food allergies should give you an indication of what is triggering your immune response. – You need to figure out which foods are causing your flare up.

## *All Chronic Diseases Starts At The Level Of A Cell*

In today's modern world we find ourselves assaulted on so many fronts at different levels from synthetic food, addiction and habitual forming substances, chemical additives and much more.

The first thing we need to understand is that the body degenerates at the level of a cell and the various disease states we see manifestations of today are simply degeneration occurring at different parts of the body. In essence your body is falling apart at different structural levels, and we classify these as different categories of diseases depending at what department of the body the chronic degeneration occurs at.

We are mislead to focus on specific components of the body when we fall ill, instead of treating ourselves holistically. After all our bodies work in harmony at the most cellular level, systems and cells communicate to each other, signaling, up regulating, etc.

The human body is composed of cells and all diseases fundamentally starts off at the cellular level before spreading to the different systems of the body. Humans are composed of trillion and trillions of cells.

From a simplistic stand point the body can be broken down into two things, cells and the extra cellular matrix. Thus, in order to understand the degenerative disease process, we need to understand things at the level of a cell and the matrix.

These cells we are composed of are nothing short of a miracle and contain organelles structures which are sub-compartments of operating machinery which have various functions. The outside of the cell known as the membrane works like an information chip processor and inside at the epicenter we find the blueprint known as DNA. Our cells perform incredible tasks, precision action, producing various chemicals at a methodical choreography.

I am just trying to describe to you how elaborate, complex, intricate and beautifully crafted every single human being is. The point I am trying to drive across is we are designed divinely and our bodies posses the necessary tools to function, but only need the correct raw materials. Input the wrong materials (junk foods) and you will pay dearly with the consequences of poor health.

Good health is our birth right and no doctor, surgeon, pharmacist and any other health care professional has any right over your divinely bestowed gift and birth right as a human being. We don't need to depend on this "medical model" for good health or any other authoritative figure because the truth has been right under our noses this whole time and that is we are in control!

Now I am not saying the innovations and advancement in technology, especially in regards to medicine is all wasted, no I am not saying that at all, however there is a time and a place for medical intervention, but when dealing with chronic diseases that are onset by lifestyle choices that we control – Than no doctor has any business with our health by manipulating our biochemistry with drugs, and literally butchering our human appendages.

We must understand that all chronic diseases is a by product of cell starvation (lack of nutrients), toxification (sugar and pollutants), and suffocation (lack of oxygen). So it doesn't matter what your struggling with whether it's the heart, bone, nerves, muscle, pancreas, etc all disease initially occurs at the level of the cell.

The issue with modern medicine is we focus too much on the specifics without considering the entire context. There is nothing wrong with being specific as we need to be in order to be precise, however we must not neglect the context of the situation and grasp everything holistically.

Now lets talk a little about the cellular matrix that also makes up the human body. The matrix is where all the electrical energy and bio-chemical synthesis occurs that drives all the incredible work of the cells found in our body. Thus, you can think of the matrix as the support of the cells that provides or feeds the cells with hormones, nutrients, oxygen, and anything else you can think of. -Also, the matrix is responsible for draining all the poisons and by products cells produce.

So now you understand the concept of cells and the matrix, so now I would like to now talk about how the onset of the disease process begins. The first point of break down for almost any chronic degenerative disease is at the point of your digestive system! The digestive system becomes compromised and dysfunctional thus causing a wide array of physiological distress. -Its really a cascading effect that systemically effects your entire body.

So, after your digestive system breaks down your blood sugar system goes awry and than your adrenal thyroid complex dysfunctions. The point I want to emphasize here is if you focus on correcting these three components of health, digestive system, blood sugar system, and the adrenal thyroid complex everything else will fall into place! – Simple right?

You're probably thinking right now, but what about if you have arthritis or any other chronic disease that is not directly connected to those 3 systems? There seems to be a disconnect, but, you need to understand that these 3 systems are behind all other bodily structures so wouldn't it make sense to strength these systems first in order to have a "domino effect" of good health?

Imagine your growing an apple tree, but for this tree to bear ripe healthy fruits you need to first put your focus on the ground or soil it is being planted into. You need to build the foundation right to get the desired result and in this case is the fruit. In this same manner the 3 systems interconnected to the entire body need to be functioning optimally for pristine health.

Hence, all the chronic disease states we are plagued with induced by our poor lifestyle choices can be thought to be the "leaves" being produced at the core of the entire breakdown process of these 3 systems. Now this is a profound realization because all we need to do is take corrective measures and focus on the root problem of diseases.

So to recap all this your living the typical American sedentary lifestyle, consume junk foods daily which lack nutrients, posses toxins (sugar), and poor oxygenation from our industrialized society, and  in conjunction with lack of exercise leads to obesity and is the jumping off point  of many other chronic degenerative disease states.

***Healing Strategies***

Nutrition

Oxygenation ( Deep breathing)

Rest

Exercise

Intermittent Fasting

Eliminating food toxicity


Health is so simple don't complicate things. The body needs proper nutrition, fresh oxygen, and small amounts of stress to stimulate growth via exercise, periods of rest, cleanses through fasting, and of course eliminating food poisons from our diet.

## Acne Case Study - Closing Thoughts

In a remote island called Kitava located near the province of *Paupa New Guinea* we find native inhabitants with the population density of 10,000-12,000 people. Untouched by western influence in regards to food supply, we find these people consuming diets rich in essential fats, vitamins, and minerals.

We found no prevalence of chronic ailments of the wester hemisphere, and it appears that these people don't seem to struggle with our type of degenerative disease states such as diabetes, dementia, high blood pressure, heart disease, etc. How can this be? Would you write this off as "its in their genetics" to have good health? Obviously not that is silly as genetics play a secondary role in the outcome of your health, and the primary influence on genetics is lifestyle choices.

Let's take a closer look at the case study conducted by professor *Steffan Lindeberg* who is a certified doctor (GP) and is a huge proponent of evolutionary nutrition. Over the course of 800+ days no signs of acne were reported in any of the population! Acne is such a common problem here in the western world and can be considered a disease of the industrialized world.

Absolutely none of the population suffered from the chronic skin disease known as acne that plagues the western world. – And there was no magic fruit or pill that they took which gave them clear skin and good health. However, their diets consisted of fish, coconuts, some fruits, yams, and other vegetables. In other words, the people of Kitava consumed *"wholefoods"* and these foods were not processed or altered by chemicals but are completely natural. – Their diets have not changed since the time of their native first generation ancestors.

They had generations upon generations of smooth and clear skin and no reports of other chronic disease states either simply because their lifestyle choices. The interesting thing is when the western diet was introduced to the populace, then only acne started to emerge and surface!

Again, we see the correlation between chronic diseases and the standard American western diet. Wholefoods vs refined foods and at this point its undisputable to even conceive you can't use wholefoods or even fasting as medicine. Simply changing your diet to a wholefood primarily plant based one can prevent chronic degenerative diseases.

## Chapter 3: Why Wholefoods Are Beneficial?

In this chapter I will discuss the importance of wholefoods, why they're beneficial to us, and 30 recommended wholefoods and delicious recipes you can try yourself.

But before I do that I wanted to ask a question, have you noticed that most major supermarkets carry almost no "wholefoods"? Most of their shelves are stocked with refined foods that can be found inside a cardboard box with mostly empty calories. This is because refined foods have longer shelf lives and last for extended periods of times because they have removed all the raw, whole, and fresh natural ingredients.

The thing about wholefoods is that although they are a powerhouse for essential vitamins and minerals, however, since they are fresh foods they don't last as long as refined foods. Now from a business stand point of view and perspective wholefoods would be a liability because you can't make as much money with foods that perish and don't last as long.

This is partly the reason why food manufacturers develop refined foods with preservatives and other additives to keep food's lifespan extended so they can sell to us the consumer and make more profits.

Wholefoods are the perfect food they contain the perfect balance and are the most nutritionally dense foods we can find on the planet. The issue is due to modern day agriculture and mineral depleted soil supply we are left with foods that lack the proper nutrition. That's not to say wholefoods cannot be produce they certainly can be, however the majority of farmers have to use additives to maintain its value.

As you know there are many minerals and vitamins that wholefoods contain. The chief among them is vitamin C which is essential to our very existence. Vitamin C is used for a myriad of biochemical functions and best of all you cannot overdose on it because its water soluble. Animals in the wild make their own vitamin C! – Humans, guerrillas and guinea pigs are the only known species who cannot produce their own vitamin C within their bodies.

The early European settlers upon arriving to North America were plagued with a disease known as scurvy. This was a nasty disease that literally made you fall apart, classical hallmark signs of scurvy are gingivitis, anemia, sore joints, and degeneration of collagen. Native aboriginals of the land introduced a remedy which was by boiling the leaves and bark of trees into an elixir and served it to the European settlers who suffered from scurvy.

Guess what? – They were cured! There disease started to reverse as soon as they drank the concoction, and surprise, surprise the reason this happened is because the leaves and tree barks that were boiled into drinks contained vitamin C! (ascorbic acid) Again, history has shown us how using nutrition as medicine is a viable treatment option to chronic diseases, and case in point that most degenerative diseases at the core are actually nutritional deficiencies! – Not random or solely "genetic" causes.

Therefore, let this be a lesson to us here in the 21st century and take this experience from the early European settlers and apply it to our lives. What if chronic diseases at the core were the result of nutritional deficiencies that manifested as bodily breakdown. Remember a chronic disease is a breakdown of the body due to poor lifestyle choices and is different from an external bacterial or viral disease.

So, we know that nutrition can help strengthen the body and reverse chronic diseases, but why do we neglect it in today's modern medicine even though history shows us otherwise? Why do we look to only solve short term symptoms neglecting the root cause? Who's vested interest does it serve to keep the masses perpetually ill?

-Imagine the amount of pharmacies and even hospitals that would go out of business if they endorsed wholefoods and an active lifestyle? I will leave it to your imagination to formulate your own answer as I have provided you all the necessary info to help you make an informed decision.

## Plant Based Foods

So what exactly are wholefoods? Well generally speaking wholefoods are plants based foods that are raw and minimally processed. Primarily vegetables is where you want to get your main source of wholefoods leafy greens, beets, bell peppers, cucumbers, cabbage, carrots, and you can even add spices or dressing to enhance flavor.

Fruits are also considered whole foods, but you got to be careful with fruits because they do contain sugar, thus eating fruits in minimal amounts along side vegetables is ok. A lot of advocates of nutrition recommend whole grain foods, but if you read this far into the book you can imagine why I do not recommend whole grain foods. – The only exception to this rule is brown rice, but again in minimal amounts too.

If we look at animals in the wild whether guerillas or elephants we observe extremely powerful creatures, yet they're diets consist of plant based foods! – Now I am not endorsing you don't need meat, but the case and point I am trying to establish is such majestic and powerful creatures in the wild consume whole foods that consist of a plant based diet.

Do we see these wild animals plagued with chronic diseases like us humans here in the industrialized world? We don't see obese, diabetic or any other form of chronic disease effecting animals in the wild, yet humans despite the great strides in our technological advancements and industrial feats still struggle with common health problems at alarming rates.

Thus, it makes sense when we see these almost miraculous results of disease reversal when patients are put on a plant based diet. People go off their insulin medication, lowers cholesterol, stabilizes blood sugar levels, blood pressure normalizes, weight loss and many other chronic symptoms reverse.

The old adage proves to be true "you are what you eat", but more specifically are what you absorb. Now I don't only endorse strictly eating plants although that is a healthy option, but I am a firm believer of balance, and you need a good source of protein from lean unprocessed meats. My top two picks are wild Alaskan Salmon and lean chicken breast, preferably organic. I know organic meat can get expensive, but even the lean meat found at grocery stores is better alternative than processed and red meats which are responsible for many chronic diseases you find at your local supermarket.

From anti-oxidants, plant phyto-nutrients, vitamins, essential fats and minerals there is no reason why you shouldn't incorporate wholefoods into your diet. The mounting scientific body of evidence cannot be disputed of the enormous health benefits and preventive measures whole foods provide. You reduce the risk of cancer, obesity, diabetes, high blood pressure and almost any other chronic degenerative disease you can think of.

Support for wholefoods primarily plant based diets is given by the *American Cancer Society*, American College of Cardiology, Harvard School of Public Health, and *the National Institute of Health.* As you can see I am not the only advocate for wholefoods as a method of prevention from the many chronic diseases that assails us in today's modern world.

## *Animal Agriculture*

As you know I am not a huge proponent of a strictly "vegan diet" without any traces of animal product, however I would like to address the fundamental issue at hand. I do endorse balanced amount of protein from whey protein powder, and a balanced amount of animal meat such as salmon to acquire your essential fatty acids. Most of your meals should be wholefoods that are plant based and there's nothing wrong with having some meat as a side, as long as you keep it proportional to vegetables and fruits.

But there is a growing concern of animal agriculture and our methods of mass producing animals to be slaughtered for the general public's consumption. In particular beef and pork, which I might add are not very healthy meat choices. You see the mass production of these types of meats through raising these animals has had some serious environmental impacts and ramifications.

Animal agriculture has contributed to more than 50% of green house gas emissions and has been associated with being the primary cause of species and habitat loss due to deforestation for grazing and growing feed crops. In America this has directly impacted our water supply with pollution and continues to dismantle our blue and pristine earth rapidly.

Thus, shifting from a primarily plant based diet will not only have a positive impact on your health, but the environment as well! You not only become a better version of yourself, but you also contribute to making the planet a better place. Now I am not going all judgemental on you or being a "animal extremist", however I am giving you some food for thought and its something to think about. I don't believe in truly cutting out all meats as we do need some substances from meat that most plants can't provide adequately, and also the fact that animals in the wild eat each other for survival too.

What I am trying to do is paint the picture of balance and harmony, so you can equip yourself with the knowledge necessary to participate in healthy eating habits.

### *What is the Ketogenic Diet?*

There is this buzzword being thrown around in the health and fitness industries known as the "ketogenic diet". But what exactly is the ketogenic diet and how is it beneficial to our health?

The ketogenic diet is a high fat, moderate protein and low carb diet. Consisting of 60-80% fat, 10-20% carbs and 20-25% protein in your diet. The key here is to create an environment that induces fat burning by having readily available fuel by burning fat present within your body with minimal carbs and moderate protein. This forces your body to switch from sugar burning to fat burning.

You ideally want to become a fat burner because if you were to compare it gram for gram in regards to fuel burning fat is superior because it's a lot cleaner. Don't believe me? Ok, well have you ever tried cooking with sugar? When its heated it leaves behind a sticky, crusty, caramel and hard to clean residue. – Now imagine this occurring in your body when you use sugar as fuel.

Fat on the other hand doesn't leave this kind of residue and burns more efficiently. Our body's sugar burning process creates something called "advanced glycated end products" also known as *AGES*.

You can consider sugar to be a dirty fuel that leaves residue behind and destruction in its wake. So, what's special about burning fat? Well, for one when you start utilizing fat for fuel you produce these molecules called "ketones", and the ongoing process of burning ketones is known as ketosis.

Ketones are high energy compounds and very easy for the body to use from brain, muscle, heart, and even for the liver. It's so ironic how we have conditioned ourselves through misinformation that fats in our diets make us fat, and although this can be true for saturated and trans-fats, but not in the case of healthy fats. It seems really counter intuitive that eating fat can help us lose weight, but the actual fact is that fat induces "fat burning" mechanisms within our bodies.

The mainstream media's way of thinking is low fat and high carbs, and this is what they promote you should be eating, but this is fundamentally erroneous on a biological scale and for the purpose of weight loss. Thus, remember the more fat you eat in the presence of low carbs, and moderate protein will enable you switch from sugar burning to fat burning.

Already you can see the multiple benefits of the ketogenic diet, cleaner source of fuel, lose weight, and have more energy to utilize!

## Difference between Paleo & Ketogenic Diet

Also known as the caveman "diet" the Paleo diet is a high protein diet, moderate fat, and low carb regiment. It is similar to the ketogenic diet but has switched the focus on high protein as oppose to high fat. Now both these diets are extremely effective for losing weight and both these regiments understand the concept of keeping your consumption of carbs low, especially refined carbs.

However, I prefer the ketogenic diet over the paleo diet. Why? Simply because with the paleo diet's focus on high protein this can potentially cause problems. As you know protein in large quantities if not utilized via exercise also converts into sugar!

Who should go on the ketogenic diet? I recommend anyone and everyone to go onto this diet because of its multiple benefits and most importantly how it forces the body to shift its metabolic process from burning sugar to fat burning. I truly believe this is the way humans are designed to eat because the body prefers using ketones and deriving your energy from sugar can cause problematic issues.

The ketogenic diet is arguably one of the best lifestyle changes to make it has anti-cancer, anti-aging, anti-seizure and many more benefits to it.

So, I've spoken a lot about fat being good for you. But what exactly is the type of fats you need to be eating? When I say fats, I am not referring to the French fries, saturated, trans fat, and hydrogenated fats. When I refer to fats I am talking about eggs, lard, butter, cheese, fish, yogurt, and organ meats. When selecting fats, you got to ensure they are minimally processed, not cooked, and are whole fats.

## *Malabsorption problems*

What if you have malabsorption problems and want to go on the ketogenic diet? You will need to start repairing the digestive system by incorporating digestive enzymes, bile salts, apple cider vinegar, lecithin, amino acids arginine, taurine, probiotics and fermented foods.

The malabsorption of fats is actually a common problem people face today in the industrialized world.

## *Theories – Evolutionary Nutrition or Fundamental Nutrition*

There are different bodies of prevailing ideologies that govern the nutrition and diet industry and even the health and fitness industry for that matter. I am going to touch on two leading philosophies which are evolutionary nutrition and fundamental nutrition. -I am not here to say one is better than the other, but the purpose of this assertion is to inform you, so you can have two different perspectives and formulate your own answers.

What is evolutionary nutrition? The premise of this ideology is that we are constantly evolving and changing, thus what we consume is destined to change over the course of time depending on selective traits we breed and influences we are exposed too. There is no absolute diet, but adaptation is the key to this theory. The assumption here is our human body's have not yet reached their prime evolution, thus we are subject to change as time progresses. Another assumption is that since our ancestors initially only started eating plant-based foods and decades later incorporated meat, then we are subject to continually evolve within the timeline.

How about the fundamental nutrition philosophy encompassing diets such as Paleo? Better known as the caveman diet, and I gravitate towards this ideology and train of thought myself. Rewinding the clock and figuring out how our ancestors ate is key to finding the right diet. The framework behind this is since there was no advanced agriculture or refining processes apart from perhaps cooking meat, our ancestors were exposed to wholefoods!

Therefore, wholefoods which are primarily plant based is what should consist of our diets. The mounting body of scientific evidence we see today is undisputable in regard to wholefood diets used to reverse chronic ailments and promote weight loss. – Thus, we don't need to keep changing our diets, but find the right type of foods with the right nutritional profile because our bodies are designed to utilize these nutritional elements as fuel.

## Chapter 4: Identify Your Body Type (Women)

You see the fact is not everybody has the same genetics, and therefore what works for them specifically may not necessarily work for you. We are all unique individuals who posses different physical traits, and to follow a generic work-out routine and expect to get shredded within a week is not realistic.

Thus, in this chapter I wanted to cover exercise routines and body types to give you a grasp of the entire picture of health and wellness. Although diet is fundamental to weight loss it works even betters and its effects are amplified in conjunction to exercise.

I've taken the liberty to give you a specifically designed exercise regiment for your precise body type. All you have to is identify your body type through the criteria I provided and follow the regiment catered towards you.

1) **Ectomorph** – lean and lanky, has difficulty building muscle, high metabolism and has a tendency to remain slender.
2) **Endomorph-** Bigger body composition, high body fat, pear shape liked, and has tendency to store fat.
3) **Mesomorph-** The more favorable body type. Naturally muscular, and posses responsive muscle cells.

(1) The Ectomorph characterized by long extremities in specific their arms and legs. These individuals tend to have a hard time gaining weight and building muscle and are noted for having slender builds. They don't have to be extremely picky on what they eat since their metabolism burns fat really quickly. – But keep this in context. Any poor eating habits can eventually lead to obesity. -Work out consists of heavier weights and less reps.

***Ectomorph Exercises:***

Stretch 2mins

Barbell Bench Press 4 sets, 4-8 reps, no more than 8 reps

Incline Dumbbell Press   4 sets, 4-8 reps, no more than 8 reps

Lying Triceps Press. 2 sets, 6-10 reps

Dumbbell Flyes. 3 sets, 10 reps.

(2) If your reading this book you probably fall into the category of endomorph. Having higher body fat composition and a tendency to store fat. Thus, losing weight is your main priority before building muscle. If you lose weight to FAST you could potentially get a condition called "loose skin", therefore do things in moderation. DO NOT rush. Loose skin is caused by

loosing huge amounts of weight (100+ lb) in a short timeframe, and this creates disfiguring skin flaps. This usually happens when people do weight loss surgery as oppose to going the natural route, but there are some instances where people have gotten loose skin due to extremely fast weight loss through working out. – Workout routine consist of rapid burst and short periods of rests, high intensity interval training.

The intention here is doing as much workout reps as possible during a set time period.

**Endomorph Exercises:**

*Cardio run/cycling at your fastest pace 5 mins. 15 second rest.*

Stretch 2mins

Squat with overhead press 1 min workout. 15 second rest.

Plank with triceps extension (dumbbells) 1 min. 15 second rest.

Push-ups 35 seconds. 15 seconds rest.

Triceps extension 45 seconds. 15 second rest.

Lunges 1 min. 15 second rest.

Jumping Jacks 1min. 15 second rest.

Side plank rotation 50 seconds. 15 second rest.

Burpees 50 seconds. 15 seconds rest.

Commandos 50 seconds. 15 second rest.

Jump squats 50 seconds. 15 second rest.

(3)Mesomorph is the most desired and favorable body type sought out after bodybuilders and athletes alike. Most athletes fall into the mesomorph continuum, and this particular body type excels extremely well in most main stream sports because of its natural muscular build and dexterity that allows individuals to move quickly and be agile. Work outs consist of moderate to high intensity interval training and short rest periods.

**Mesomorph Exercises:**

Stretch 2 mins

Barbell Bench Press 4 sets, 8-12 reps

Dumbbell Flyes. 3 sets, 12-14 reps.

Incline Dumbbell Press   4 sets, 8-10 reps

Ab crunches  3 sets , 25 reps

Push ups 3 sets, 20 reps

Barbell deadlift  2 sets 6 reps

Pec dec   3 sets 20 reps

Pull ups 2 sets do as much as you can

Bicep curls 2 sets 25 reps

Squats 2 sets 20 reps

## *Importance of Gut Health – Probiotics*

The gut can be considered your second brain and is where the majority of cells that make up your immune system are found. The entire digestive system has an important role to play in our health ranging from the immune system, central nervous system, skin, blood pressure and cardiovascular health.

The digestive system is composed of the stomach, small and large intestines, and other accessory organs. I want to specifically talk about the intestines as this is where the "good bacteria" are found. If you live anywhere in North America or any industrialized society for that matter, chances are you have poor gut health due to the wear and tear you've assaulted your body with from your lifestyle choices. From refined foods, alcohol, pollution, antibiotics etc. You probably have a form of dysbiosis. -Dysbiosis is just a fancy way of saying you have an imbalance of bacteria in your intestines.

Dysbiosis can manifest in many different forms such as asthma, ear infections, excess mucous production in nose or throat, and even acne. When our gut is out of whack it creates a domino effect throughout every major system in the body. Thus, the importance of keeping our microbiome healthy because its responsible for various important physiological functions in our body such as communicating with other cells, digestive processes, and detoxification of heavy metals, food toxins and hormones by products.

Hence, I stress the importance of consuming foods rich in probiotics too. Fermented food is where you can find loads of probiotics and fiber which will aid in the repair and strengthening of your microbiome. The key to restoring gut health is *1*. Eliminate food toxins *2*. Use multiple strains of good bacteria *3*. Consume more fiber.

## *Chapter 5: 30 Whole Foods & Recipes*

The whole premise of this book is eating less calories and periods of fasting in conjunction to whole foods and exercise will increase the likelihood of weight loss, prevent chronic degenerative diseases, and promote health and wellness.

I've discussed everything from fasting and the science behind it, and the intricate biochemistry behind our body's blueprint, insidious marketing ploys by food manufactures and corporations, and the powerful benefits of wholefoods.

Now this is probably the moment you been waiting for as one of the primary reasons you purchased this book was to learn about *magic 30 wholefoods* that will help you with weight loss! Now remember I don't guarantee you will lose 30 pounds in a month like some of my avid readers have experienced, but I am more than certain you will have some degree of success with your weight loss journey when you implement all my strategies.

Without further ado lets get into the special 30 wholefoods you need for weight loss and some nutritious recipes too. Below is provided my must have list of whole foods, bonus flavor enhancing ingredients, fermented foods and healthy recipes to follow:

## 30 Wholefoods

Nutritional Yeast

Oysters

Eggs (preferably boiled or raw)

Sprouts

Avocado

Salmon

Herring

Halibut

Algae

Olives

Chickpeas (rinse and drained)

Green & red bell peppers

Cucumbers

Tomatoes

Onions

Spinach

Strawberries

Blueberries

Pineapples

Romanian Cabbage

Almonds

Sunflower seeds

Pumpkin seeds

Chicken breast

Brown rice

Squash

Papaya

Cauliflower

Broccoli

Mushrooms

Kale & Zucchini

*All the above mentioned foods are an excellent source of*

**Vitamins:** *C, D, A, E, K, H, B complex (B1-B12)*

**Macro Minerals:** *Calcium, Phosphorus, Magnesium, Potassium, and Sodium*

***Trace Minerals:*** *Selenium, Chromium, Vanadium, Iron, Zinc, Copper, Fluoride, and Iodide*

***Essential Fatty Acids****: Omega 3,6 & 9*

## Bonus  Ingredients/Supplements

Olive oil

Sesame seed oil

Coconut oil

Whey protein

Casein protein powder

Hemp protein powder

Pea protein powder

Egg white protein powder

Salt

Pepper

Paprika

Mint

Clove

Oregano

Parsley

Cinnamon

Lemon juice

Lime juice

### *Fermented Foods – Restoring Gut Health*

**Kefir** - fermented milk drink made with a yeast/bacterial fermentation starter of kefir grains.

**Kimchi** - Originates from Korean cuisine, made from salted and fermented vegetables, most commonly napa cabbage and Korean radishes, with a variety of seasonings, including scallions, garlic, and ginger.

**Natto** - made from soybeans fermented with Bacillus subtilis.

**Tempeh** - Is made by a natural culturing and controlled fermentation process that binds soybeans into a cake form.

**Miso** - produced by fermenting soybeans with salt and koji and sometimes rice, barley, seaweed or other ingredients.

**Pickles** – Cucumber that has been pickled in a brine, vinegar, or other solution and left to ferment for a period of time

**Sauerkraut** - Raw cabbage that has been fermented by various lactic acid bacteria

**Kombucha** - Fermented tea that is slightly alcoholic.

All the above mentioned ingredients from 30 whole foods to fermented foods contain all if not most the vitamins, minerals, probiotics, and essential fatty acids you require for optimal health. These are the major components and building blocks to good health and I strongly urge you to incorporate most of these listed ingredients into your diets in conjunction with fasting plus exercise and you will see amazing results within 3-4 weeks if you follow the regiment consistently.

## 33 Recipes

### 1.Keto Cabbage Stir Fry

Ingredients

- 20 oz. green cabbage
- 3-5 oz. butter
- 20 oz. ground beef or chicken
- 2 tsp salt
- 2 tsp onion powder
- ¼ tsp ground black pepper
- 2 tbsp white wine vinegar
- 3 garlic cloves
- 1 tsp chili flakes
- 1 tbsp fresh ginger, finely chopped or grated
- 1 tbsp sesame oil

### *2. Keto Fried Chicken*

Ingredients

- 2 lbs boneless chicken thighs
- 3-5 oz. butter
- 1 lb broccoli
- ½ leek
- 2 tsp garlic powder
- salt and pepper (optional )

### 3. Keto Scrambled Eggs

Ingredients

- 1 oz. butter
- 2 eggs
- salt and pepper
- 1 tbsps olive oil
- Hand full of green & green peppers
- Dash of Coriander

### 4. Keto Style Pizza

Ingredients

**Crust**

- 4-6 eggs
- 6 oz. shredded cheese, preferably mozzarella

**Topping**

- 3-5 tbsp tomato paste
- 1 tsp dried oregano
- 5 oz. shredded cheese
- 2 oz. pepperoni
- Black & Green Olives

**For serving**

- 5 oz. leafy greens
- 4 tbsp olive oil
- salt and pepper
- Hand full of green & green peppers
- Dash of Coriander

### 5. Keto Chicken Bowl

Ingredients

- 10 oz. Romaine lettuce
- 5 oz. cherry tomatoes
- 3 avocados
- 3 tbsp fresh cilantro
- 3-5 oz. butter
- 1½ lbs boneless chicken thighs
- salt and pepper
- 2 yellow onion
- 2 green bell pepper
- 5 oz. cheese

### 6. Keto chicken & Eggs

- 6 eggs scrambled
- Green & red bell peppers
- Onions
- 2 chicken breast  (well cooked)
- cherry tomatoes (optional)
- fresh parsley (optional)

### 7. Keto Salad

Ingredients

- 4 oz. celery stalks
- 2 scallions
- 5 oz. tuna in olive oil
- ¾ cup mayonnaise
- ½ lemon, zest and juice
- 2 tsp Dijon mustard
- 4 eggs
- ½ lb Romaine lettuce
- 4 oz. cherry tomatoes
- 2 tbsp olive oil
- salt and pepper

### 8. Keto Salmon Biscuit

Ingredients

- 4 oz heavy cream
- 8 oz cream cheese spread
- 2 oz cheddar cheese
- 8 oz provolone cheese
- 3 eggs

## DRIED HERBS & SPICES

- Oregano
- Cayenne Pepper
- Red pepper flakes (optional)
- Pepper
- Sea salt

*9. Meat & Seed Feast*

## FISH

- 6-8 oz smoked salmon

## FRUIT AND VEG

- 1 red bell pepper
- 1 red onion
- 1 onion
- 2 lemon
- 2 green onion (spring onion)
- 1 broccoli
- 6 oz lettuce
- 3 oz cherry tomatoes
- Lime
- 3 oz mushrooms
- 2 jalapenos
- 2 bell peppers
- 1 bag arugula

## MEAT

1 lb chicken thigh, with skin and bone

## NUTS, SEEDS, WHOLEFOODS

- 3 oz chia seeds
- 8 oz sesame seeds

## OILS, FATS

- 6 fl oz olive oil
- 1 fl oz sesame oil
- 1 fl oz coconut oil
- 3 oz peanut butter

## SAUCES, CONDIMENTS

- 4 fl oz soy sauce (low sodium)

## BAKING

- 1 3/4 tbsp coconut flakes
- 2 1/2 tsp cocoa powder
- Vanilla extract
- 2 oz almond flour
- 5 tsp stevia
- 1 tsp baking powder

### Sesame mayonnaise

- 1 egg yolk, at room temperature
- 1 tsp Dijon mustard
- ½ cup avocado oil or light olive oil
- 1 tbsp sesame oil
- ½ tbsp lime juice
- salt and pepper

## Salad

- 2 scallions
- 3 oz. cherry tomatoes
- 2 oz. cucumber
- 3 oz. lettuce
- ½ red onion
- fresh cilantro
- 1 tbsp sesame seeds

### 10. Keto Pesto Chicken

Ingredients

- 25 oz. chicken thighs or chicken breasts
- 2 oz. butter, for frying
- 3 oz. red pesto or green pesto
- 1½ cups heavy whipping cream
- ½ cup pitted olives
- 8 oz. feta cheese, diced
- 1 garlic clove, finely chopped
- salt and pepper (optional )

### 11. Keto Oven Baked Salmon

Ingredients

- 4-6 oz salmon
- Butter
- Handful of Broccoli
- 2 Tbsp Salt and pepper

### *12. Keto Chicken Salad*

Ingredients

- 1 tablespoon red wine vinegar
- 3 cups of kale
- 1 cup shredded cabbage
- 3 cups of sliced tomatoes
- 3 avocados
- 6-8 8 oz cooked chicken oven baked

### 13. Chick Pea Salad

- 1 can of chicken peas ( rinsed and drained)
- 1 cucumber chopped
- 2 Tomatoes
- ½ diced onion
- 1 Tbsp of Olive oil
- Handful of parsley or mint
- Salt & pepper
- ½ red or green bell peppers
- ½ cup of sunflower seeds

### 14. *Fruit & Veggie Smoothie*

- Water
- 5oz Spinach
- Strawberries (frozen)
- Mango (frozen )
- 2 Bananas

### 15. *Rice & Garlic Chicken*

- ½ brown rice
- 2 cups of chick peas (rinse and drained)
- 2 tbsp of salt & pepper
- 2 tbsp of olive oil
- 1 lb of chicken
- ½ diced onions

### 16. *Vegan Soup*

- 2 Sweet potatoes
- ½ lb cauliflower
- 1 lb carrots
- Pinch of salt

*Instructions:  Boil all ingredients in pot of water. Than drain residue, keep content and blend everything in blender until creamy thickness. - Add a handful of sunflower seeds for crunch texture after soup is produced. ( optional)

### 17. Coconut Salmon

- 1 Salmon
- 2 tbsp Sesame seeds
- 1 tbsp of coconut butter
- Handful of shredded coconut
- Tbsp of olive oil
- Pinch of Salt
- 3 cups of steamed broccoli with butter
- Pinch or Parsley

### 18. *Spicy & Roasted Chickpeas*

- 2 cans of chickpeas rinsed and drained (bake chickpeas 350 Fahrenheit for 20 mins)
- Garlic powder
- Paprika
- Ginger
- Salt
- Pepper
- Turmeric
- Olive oil
- Mix with Avocado

### 19. Healthy Pudding

- Cup of Diced Almonds
- 2 Bananas
- Shredded coconut
- Almond milk
- 1 tbsp of stevia extract
- 2 tbsp of chia seeds (optional)

*Instructions: Blend all ingredients together until creamy and than store in fridge overnight.

## 20. Egg Salad

- 2 Diced hard boiled egg
- Pinch of salt and pepper
- Green & Red peppers diced 1 tbsp
- ½ Dijon mustard
- 2 celery stalks chopped
- Pinch of paprika

*Instructions:  Mix all ingredients in a bowl and ready to serve.

### 21. Masala

- Chickpeas rinse and drained
- 2 ½   Brown rice
- 1 tbsp of olive oil ( or coconut oil)
- 2 tbsp of masala seasoning
- ½   salt & pepper
- ½   diced onion
- 2 chilli peppers
- 1/3 tomato sauce
- Pinch of turmeric
- 1 cup of vegetable broth
- Pinch of parsley

## 22. Fruit Salad

- ½  cup of grapes
- 3 kiwi diced
- Pinch of lemon juice
- 2 mangos diced
- ½  pomegranates arils
- 5 orange slices

### 23. Pomegranate Smoothie

- 2 frozen bananas
- ½ chopped pears
- 1/3 pomegranate juice
- 1/3 Almond milk

*Instructions: mix all ingredients and blend well. Ready to serve right away.

### 24. Sweet Dijon Chicken Rice Bowl

- 2 ½   of brown rice (cooked)
- 2 boneless chicken breasts
- 2 avocados
- 1/3 Maple syrup
- Dijon Mustard
- ½ cup of sesame seeds
- Pinched of shredded coconut

### 25. BBQ Chicken Rice Bowl

- 2 boneless chicken breasts
- 2 avocados
- Diced pineapples
- BBQ sauce

## 26. Tuna Salad

- Canned Tuna
- 1 avocado
- Salt & pepper
- 1 tbsp Olive oil
- 2 tbsp lemon juice

### 27. Chili

- 1 each of red and black beans (rinsed and drained)
- 1 boneless chicken breast diced
- Bowl of quinoa
- 2 tbsp of chilli powder
- ½ cup of diced onions
- Salt & pepper
- Pinch of paprika
- Pinch of cumin
- Parsley
- 1 diced tomato

### 28. Strawberry Slushy

- 4-6 basil leaves
- 2½ cups of frozen strawberry
- Choose either lemon or lime juice 1/3 ( 3 lemons or limes – *pick one*)

### 29. Avocado Salad

- 2 diced avocados
- ½ lemon juice
- 1 diced tomato
- Handful of Romanian cabbage
- Salt and pepper
- Olive oil

### 30. Tofu Rice Bowl

- 1.5 cup of brown rice
- 3 tbsp of soya sauce
- 1 diced avocado
- Tofu (marinated)
- Green bell peppers
- Salt and pepper
- Handful of mushrooms

### How to marinate Tofu

- 1 Tbsp garlic sauce
- 1 tbsp of soya sauce
- Olive oil
- Salt and pepper (optional)

### 31. *Classic* BBQ chicken & Vegetables

- 1 pound (lb) of boneless chicken breast
- 1.5 cups of sweet potatoes
- 1 cup of steam broccoli
- 1 cup of steam asparagus
- Chilli powder
- BBQ sauce ( Trader Joe's Kansas City BBQ Sauce)
- Salt and pepper

### 32. Brown Rice & Garlic Chicken Bowl

- 1.5 cups of brown rice
- 2 cups of chickpeas (rinse and drained)
- ½ lb of broccoli
- 5 oz of spinach
- 1 garlic (pressed into paste)
- 1 lb of boneless chicken breast
- Salt and pepper
- 1 tbsp of olive oil
- 2 cups of water

### 33. Coconut Curry Rice Bowl

- 1 tbsp of curry powder
- 1 diced tomato
- 2 dice sweet potatoes
- Salt and pepper
- Pinch of parsley
- 1.5 cup of brown rice
- ½ chopped onion
- Coconut milk (1 can)

### Conclusion

Congratulation you've reached the end of the book! You've learned quite a lot and now its time for you to start implementing everything you have learnt and start seeing results!

Remember to pace yourself and increase your fasting periods in incremental steps, also use the recipes and my choice wholefoods listed in conjunction with exercise to achieve maximum results.

You've learned everything from the dark secretes of food manufactures designing habit forming foods, intermittent fasting, mindful eating, chronic degenerative diseases, benefits of wholefoods, exercise regiments, bio-hacks, body types and even a little bio-chemistry.

You have everything you need to equip yourself on your weight loss journey. Feel free to write to me at info@healthypslife.com if you have any further inquires. I am more than willing to help you where I can. Remember you are not alone in this journey and can reference this resource at any point in time if your feeling stuck or need motivation.

I trust you are on your way to becoming the greatest version of yourself you just need to follow through. This is *Ashley Dawnson* wishing you a happy life full of abundance, longevity, peace of mind, health and wellness.

If you need food journals you can check out my author profile on amazon, which has two neat food journals you can use to keep things neat, accountable and measure your progress. (Or see below)

Food journal 1: https://amzn.to/2QcKoYS

Food journal 2: https://amzn.to/2AJupfI

I wish you the best on your journey, feel free to message me on your progress, updates or even your personal struggles.

Sincerely,

Ashley Dawnson

## *Glossary*

***Addiction*** - habitual forming habits that become perpetual and uncontrollable causing conflict within our willpower on both a physiological and psychological level.

***Artificial Sweeteners*** – substitutes or substances that are used in place of sugar.

***Anti-Aging*** - reversing the degeneration process externally and internally.

***Blood Sugar Levels*** – the amount of glucose found within our blood stream at any given time.

***Carbohydrates*** – refers to leafy green vegetables and fruits as oppose to "refined carbohydrates" that encompass pasta, breads, and pastries.

***Craving*** – A built in internal drive that humans posses a particular desire for and have an appetite that panders to it.

***Cellular matrix*** – where more specialized structures are embedded and can be found.

***Euphoria*** – A feeling of elation or excitement.

***Evolutionary Nutrition*** – a philosophy that endorses that human beings are constantly evolving, and we have not stopped evolving, but continue to evolve and as such our dietary and nutritional needs will continue change over the course of time.

**Functional Eating** – Eating for our needs of survival like animals in the wild.

**Frequency** - rate at which something occurs or is repeated over a particular period of time.

**Glucose** - a simple sugar that is an important energy source in living organisms and is a component of many carbohydrates.

**Intermittent fasting** – Restricting the amount of caloric intake you have and frequency of meals during the day.

**Insulin** – Master hormone that is responsible for several biochemical functions, such as delegating fat storage and sugar burning for fuel.

**Glycogen** - a substance deposited in bodily tissues as a storage of carbohydrates. It is a polysaccharide that forms glucose on hydrolysis.

**Glucagon**- a hormone formed in the pancreas that promotes the breakdown of glycogen to glucose in the liver.

**Ghrelin** – hunger hormones responsible for hunger.

**Leptin** - satiety hormone tells us  not to eat anymore.

**MRI** – Magnetic resonance imaging; imaging technique used in radiology to form pictures of anatomy.

**Paleo diet** – known as the "cave man diet" high protein, moderate fat and low carbs.

**Parasympathetic nervous system** – Responsible for rest and relax mode.

**Refined-Carbohydrates** – Foods that have been refined and stripped of their essential nutrients, breads, pasta, white rice, white bread, etc

**Refined- Foods** - Any foods that have been refined and stripped of their essential nutrients this can be meats, carbs, and fats that have all been altered.

**Sugar Addiction** – A strong dependency and uncontrollable desire for the substance sugar which leads to a lot of health crisis and chronic degenerative diseases.

**Sympathetic nervous system-** Responsible for fight or flight mode.

Made in the USA
Columbia, SC
12 May 2019